THE 9 DECREES OF DIABETES

A SIMPLE 9 STEP PLAN TO REVERSING TYPE 2 DIABETES, HELPING YOU ACHIEVE REMISSION THROUGH FASTING, DIET AND EXERCISE AS IT HELPED ME

JONAH Y JOSEPH
DR. N GORDON

Especially

For You

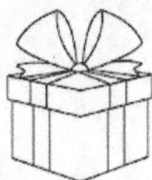

As a thank you, grab your <u>Free</u> Copy of "99 ways to lose 1 Pound Every Month While Still Eating The Foods You Love" and start your journey to remission today!

Visit the link below and enjoy

www.jonahyjoseph.com/Resources

CONTENTS

ADVANCE PRAISES

This is a highly challenging and inspirational book by Jonah Joseph on the impact of lifestyle change in reversing both pre- diabetes and type 2 diabetes. The personal experience combined with robust scientific evidence-based information provides both the motivation and a stable platform to make wise choices contributing to an abundant life. The simple, easy read information on human physiology makes it a handbook on healthy living and is a must for every household.

Dr. A. Gomez; MBBS, DPM, MRCPsych; Consultant Psychiatrist in Learning Disabilities, West Midlands.

I started reading this book by Jonah Joseph and was very pleasantly surprised by how well informed and researched the topic was. Though the author is not medically trained, he has taken a very methodical approach, quoting appropriate up-to- date references from the medical literature on diabetes and cardiovascular risk. The most remarkable thing about this book is the personal story he tells about his own journey and subsequent learning that we can all learn from.

The book is easy to read and very enjoyable and one that I would strongly recommend given the increasing prevalence of diabetes in our communities. It gives great advice for those who have pre-diabetes and diabetes and will also be invaluable to those at risk of developing this terrible disease which in many instances is preventable and reinforces the old adage that prevention is better than cure...

Professor Faizel Osman MB BCh MD FRCP FESC; Consultant Cardiologist / Electrophysiologist

Honorary Professor of Cardiology (Warwick Medical School)

Lead for Cardiac Rhythm Management Department of Cardiology

University Hospital Coventry.

The 9 Decrees of Diabetes by Jonah Joseph is an essential read for all people, especially those with prediabetes and type 2 diabetes. This book is particularly relevant when obesity and metabolic disorders contribute significantly to global morbidity and mortality. It is a brilliant resume on a range of factors from diet through to sleep that can affect insulin secretion and blood sugar levels. The dynamic content of the book, especially the chapters on diet, fasting, and exercise, should inspire all to pursue a lifestyle change.

Dr. Sheeja Cherian MSc (Biochemistry) Ph.D. (Diabetes Research); Retired Lecturer in Biomedical Sciences, Halesowen College, UK.

MY STORY

G rowing up, I was constantly reminded that "be very careful as you have Diabetes in your family."
I never really took much notice as I enjoyed my food and have a very sweet tooth which I guess most diabetics do from what I've seen.

As time went by, and when I was in my thirties, I realized that occasionally, I would get light-headed, my head would begin to feel heavy as if its weight was trying to bring me down.

I even remember having a blackout at the local library once where everything went dark for a few seconds and also getting spells of dizziness which were becoming more frequent; I never gave it much thought and put it down to me not drinking enough water, diabetes never once entered my mind.

It was in 2016 when an uncle of mine returned from abroad; knowing how much I loved sweets brought me back some made purely from sugar and ghee.

I very happily consumed the sweets, but after this, I realized that I had to see a doctor as the heaviness in my head began to worsen.

I spoke with my family, who told me to get it checked immediately because there was a history of diabetes in my family.

And so, I phoned the chemist to book an appointment for a blood glucose test.

When I phoned, they told me that to get accurate results I needed to fast from the night before, therefore, I wasn't allowed to consume anything after 8 pm which I followed and the very next day, I visited them, they did free blood and glucose tests as well as other tests.

When I arrived, I was taken into their consultation room where they carried out the tests, and after seeing the results of the test, they gave me that surprised look; I was curious; it was that look that made you impatient and makes you want to scream out, what is it! What's wrong I was thinking, have they caught something more severe than what I had imagined?

Unfortunately for me, it was not good news. The days where I could consume sweets and chocolates without having to worry were over as I was told that although I had been fasting for 12 hours by the time the test was carried out, my blood sugar levels were still reading very high.

They were concerned; they told me to see my doctor as soon as possible without delay; it was convenient that my doctor's surgery was just above the chemist. So, I immediately went upstairs and booked an appointment to see her.

When I went into the surgery, my doctor explained that as my reading was of concern and because there was a history of diabetes in my family, she would book me in for further testing at the local hospital.

After a few days, I received the appointment letter from my local hospital. They also asked me to fast from the night before as they wanted to run several further tests that were needed to see the bigger picture of what was happening with my blood glucose.

After taking the tests, they told me that my doctor would give me a call with the test results; she called me after a couple of days and broke the news to me that I have been classed as a type 2 diabetic and that I should start taking medication as soon as possible to help me with this as a matter of urgency.

She even went as far as to write down the prescriptions for the medicines that I would require and began to explain the help I could receive in paying for my medications as I would need quite a lot of different pills and would require them routinely, the cost of which would run relatively high if no help was available.

When I was a teenager, I remember very clearly when a close friend of mine once explained to me about the human immune system, what it is, how it works, and how to strengthen it by allowing it to work on its own without pills and medication, etc.

He explained to me how drugs and medicines stopped the immune system from working to its full potential and how the immune system becomes lazy.[1]

Ever since that day, I became very health conscious and refused to take any medication that I believed I could cope without unless I absolutely needed it, and till this day, I will only take one aspirin in dire and extreme circumstances, which, when taken, does work wonders for me.

This, I believe, is all due to my immune system being strong and only because I took on board what my friend explained and who I am genuinely thankful to.

I explained to my doctor that I strongly believe in the human body's power to heal and in the immune system and would like to be given a chance to see if I can do something else rather than take medicine; she took a while to think about what else they could offer me.

After a while, she told me about this educational course that was being trialed, known as DESMOND (Diabetes Education and Self-Management for Ongoing and Newly Diagnosed). She asked me if I would like to take this route and be enrolled in this course.

I immediately took up the offer, and a week later, I received the invitation letter and was off to this course.

When I arrived at the venue, I was greeted by the tutors and taken to a room filled with people of all different backgrounds and ages, all of whom had also been diagnosed like myself with diabetes.[2]

Many of the people in that room were newly diagnosed, some with type one, others type two, ladies with gestational diabetes, as well as people that had diabetes and had been taking medication for a while.

The course was laid out very well; it began with explaining about training the mindset to adapt to and accept lifestyle changes, believing that anything was possible only with willpower and if the human mind allowed and believed in it.

The entire course was structured around what we consume, our eating habits, good ones and bad, our downfalls, and what we must do to turn this around in the safest, fastest, and best way possible.

In the course, I learned that my entire life, I was making the wrong choices and decisions when it came to lifestyle choices, food, and satisfying my hunger, which led me to be diagnosed with diabetes and sitting there as a patient.

The course tutors explained what sugar and glucose were, how and what foods turned into sugars and which ones didn't, what the ideal dinner plate should look like, what measurements our servings should be, the importance of diet and losing weight, the benefits of fasting, the importance of sleep and mental health, the importance of hydration and the adverse effects of alcohol and smoking, and how all of this can be carried out in the best and safest way.

After listening to the tutors, their words touched me, as losing weight was something that I urgently needed to do as I was a very unhealthy 224 pounds (16 stone).

I used to get tired and out of breath while climbing the two flights of stairs in my home, which had also been in the back of my mind for a while now.

I used to think to myself that if my children ever asked me to play football, I wouldn't last 2 minutes without the need to sit down and take a break.

I guess it had to take being labeled a "diabetic" to give me that wake-up call as this was the only way I would understand that I needed to make positive lifestyle changes urgently.

I remember the tutors of the course saying that in the past, they have had students who, like the people in the room, were diagnosed and who had successfully put their diabetes into remission; one of those students even decided to become a tutor and help deliver the course to inspire others.

I wanted to be that person; I wanted to help others who were diagnosed; I also wanted to be the one that had successfully put their diabetes into remission, and thankfully today, I can say that five years down the line, I am still on no medication and have also lost weight and hence why I have decided to write this book to inspire you and others.

I lost so much weight that I had to change my wardrobe; this also positively impacted my confidence and helped turn my life around for the better; I went from being an unhealthy 224 pounds (16 stone) to a healthy 182 pounds (13 stone).

All of this was done only because I believed in myself because I wanted to change. After all, I wanted to live a quality life free from doctor's appointments and hospital visits.

So here I am today, continuing my journey to try and live my life as best as possible without the complications and worries that diabetes can bring and, more importantly, without the medication.

And because I am diagnosed, my name is also on the diabetes register. Therefore, I annually receive all the tests from eyesight to blood pressure and glucose tests that other diagnosed diabetics receive.

And thankfully, like every year, even this year, I was told by my diabetes clinic nurse that I have nothing to worry about as long as I continue doing what I have been, which is following all of the course information from having a disciplined diet and exercise regime to generally making the right lifestyle choices.

I don't starve myself; after all, I'm human. I also have cravings, and if you have a sweet tooth like me, you will understand that a sweet tooth never goes away. I do have cheat days where I will have something sweet the difference now is that I manage to control what I eat and how much of it, and I also know when to stop and what to do after.

How did I achieve all of this? This was due to my lifestyle changes and routine, which I adopted after taking the course; I began by making a plan on gradually losing weight over some time, realizing that consistency is the key.

I took up jogging, I started off very slowly and managed to build myself up, and I now jog 4 to 5 times a week; I'm not training to compete in the Olympics! So, I don't need to jog very fast or break any records; I just want to lose some weight, anything; even if I lose ten calories, it's a step in the right direction.

Out of the many things that I took away from the course, the one thing I remember the most from DESMOND is that if a person was to lose 100 calories a week by making small tiny changes and kept consistent over some time. The difference would be enormous; They will eventually lose weight; it may take a while, but consistency is the key, and ultimately, they will get there.

When I first began to jog, I would get tired, but instead of stopping for a break to get my breath back or stop running altogether and start walking, which most people do, I would carry on.

I wouldn't stop; I would just slow my pace right down to a very slow jogging pace almost like a speed walk, one that I am comfortable with, and the reason I did this was because I didn't want my heart rate to drop, and I wanted to keep up that sweat!

After a while, I began seeing results; it was working; I was finally losing weight and all because of those tiny little things that I had removed and also added to my daily routine; this also encouraged me to make other changes because when you see that something is working, making a difference, it gives you confidence and strength.

I introduced a fasting regime into my week and began fasting every Monday and Thursday where I would not consume anything from dawn till sunset, after which I would just have the one meal as I would on any other day; this also helped me towards my goal as I was losing weight faster, getting lighter and healthier.

This is my success story, putting my diabetes into remission and staying off the drugs purely through fasting, diet, and exercise, and I genuinely believe that if it has helped me and I can do it, then so can you!

So, if you want to put your diabetes into remission, continue reading this book to find out what I learned from the course and how you can also successfully put your diabetes into remission by making the lifestyle changes that I did.[3] 😊

1

UNDERSTANDING YOUR CONDITION

The concept of "prediabetes" is rather vague and often misunderstood. How can one have prediabetes, and what exactly is it? Surely, diabetes is a condition whereby you either have it, or you don't. Unfortunately (or fortunately, depending on one's outlook), diabetes is just not that simple as most things in life.

Prediabetes refers to a condition whereby blood sugar levels are higher than they should be but not high enough to be classed as a person who has type 2 diabetes.[1] Prediabetes consists of two clinical entities: impaired fasting glucose (IFG) and impaired glucose tolerance (IGT).[2]

It is estimated that about 88 million American adults have prediabetes-more than 84% do not know that they

have it. 84% is a relatively large number, but how does one know that they have prediabetes?

The answer is simple, prediabetes does not have apparent symptoms and therefore may go undetected for years. Without clear signs and symptoms, one needs to be aware of the risk factors associated with prediabetes.

Risk factors for the development of prediabetes include being overweight (For adults, overweight is defined as having a BMI higher than 25, and obesity is defined as having a BMI higher than 30. BMI is calculated as a person's weight (in kg) divided by the square of height (m^2)[3], being the age of 45 or over, having a parent or sibling with type 2 diabetes, living a sedentary lifestyle (being physically active less than three times per week), having a previous history of pregnancy-induced diabetes (gestational diabetes), previously giving birth to a baby weighing 9 pounds(4 kg) or more, having polycystic ovarian syndrome (Polycystic ovarian syndrome (PCOS) refers to a hormonal disorder found in a woman of reproductive age. Symptoms include irregularities in the menstrual cycle, excess facial and body hair, acne, raised blood glucose levels, and polycystic ovaries[4], and race and ethnicity.

Studies have shown that African Americans, Hispanic/Latino Americans, American Indians, Pacific Islanders, and some Asian Americans are at a higher risk of developing prediabetes than other races and ethnicities.[5]

Testing, or rather screening for prediabetes, is effortless and straightforward. And the results should be available relatively quickly. There are ranges of quick and easy tests which can be done[6]:

- **The Fasting blood glucose test.** This test measures blood glucose levels following an overnight fast.
- **The Random blood glucose test.** This test measures the blood glucose level at the time of testing. Random blood glucose testing does not require a starved or content state, hence its name "random."
- **The HbA1c/A1C test.** This measures the average glucose levels in the blood over the past two to three months. This test is a good indicator of blood glucose control, especially in patients who have overt diabetes.
- **The oral glucose tolerance test (OGTT).** This test is a bit more intricate. First, it requires an overnight fast. And then, upon presentation to the doctor, an initial fasting blood glucose reading is taken, followed by drinking a sugar-containing liquid. The blood glucose level is then re-checked and recorded at hour one, hour two, and possibly again at hour three.

The next table shows the values and ranges of the tests mentioned above and how one is classified as normoglycemic, prediabetic, or diabetic based on the values obtained from the diagnostic tests.

Result	Fasting blood glucose	Random blood glucose	A1C test	Oral glucose tolerance test
Normoglycemia	< 99mg/dL (5.49mmol/L)	N/A	Below 5.7%	< 140mg/dL (7.77mmol/L)
Prediabetes	100-125mg/dL (5.55-6.94mmol/L)	N/A	5.7-6.4%	140-199mg/dL (7.77-11.04mmol/L)
Diabetes	>126mg/dL (6.99mmol/L)	> 200mg/dL (11.1mmol/L)	> 6.5%	> 200mg/dL (11.1mmol/L)

Table 1: showing the results of diagnostic tests for normoglycemia, prediabetes, and diabetes.[7]

Once one has been diagnosed with prediabetes, the next natural step in managing prediabetes is understanding how one develops prediabetes.

Insulin resistance is synonymous with prediabetes. This is because body tissues, especially the muscles, become resistant to the effects of insulin. This results in less glucose being taken up by the body tissues, ultimately leading to a high glucose concentration in the blood.

With a sustained increase in blood glucose levels, there is increased secretion of insulin from the pancreas. However, over time, the pancreas is unable to cope with the increased demand for insulin in Susceptible individuals.

Eventually, the pancreas cells become exhausted and can no longer secrete insulin- this is known as Beta-cell failure (B-cell failure). The key feature here is that there is a relative insulin deficiency.

In other words, there is insufficient insulin production to overcome the tissue's resistance rather than absolute insulin deficiency.[8]

And if this process continues and is allowed to go on without intervention, there is a high chance that ultimately prediabetes will evolve into type 2 diabetes.

The Diabetes Prevention Program (DPP), a large long-term study, found that by adopting a healthy diet and lifestyle, prediabetes and ultimately the onset of type 2 diabetes can be prevented.

The study involved 3,234 participants. All of the participants were overweight and had impaired glucose tolerance (IGT). In addition, 45% of the participants were from races or ethnicities, which are associated with a higher incidence of diabetes (African American, Hispanic American/Latino, Asian American or Pacific Islander, and American Indian).

The participants were then divided into three groups. The first group received intensive training in diet, exercise, and behavior modification.

The second group was given an oral hypoglycemic drug (metformin 850mg) to take twice a day. And the third group received placebo medication instead of oral hypoglycemic drugs.

The second and third groups also received training on diet and exercise but not intense counseling on it.

Now, the participants in group 1 reduced their risk of developing diabetes by 58%. Lifestyle changes showed that the best results were for those participants over the age of 60; their risk was reduced by 71%.

The participants in group 2 reduced their risk of developing diabetes by 31%, and the metformin was less effective in reducing the risk of diabetes in those aged over 45 years.

However, metformin was most effective in participants aged between 25-44 years and those with a BMI lower than 35. About 5% of participants in group 1 developed diabetes each year during the study period, about 7.8% in group 2 and 11% in group 3.[9]

The participants in group 1 (who showed the most significant risk reduction in developing diabetes) were given 16 classes teaching them basic nutrition and behavioral strategies for weight loss and physical activity, lifestyle coaches, supervised physical activity sessions, and constant reinforcement.[10]

NOW, IF PREDIABETES IS THE PRECURSOR TO TYPE 2 DIABETES, WHAT EXACTLY IS TYPE 2 DIABETES?

Well, type 2 diabetes refers to a clinical entity characterized by variable degrees of insulin resistance,

impaired insulin secretion, and excessive glucose production by the liver.[11]

The underlying mechanism for the development of type 2 diabetes is the same as prediabetes. However, the difference between prediabetes and type 2 diabetes is that the underlying process, which allows for the development of prediabetes, is allowed to continue, ultimately resulting in type 2 diabetes.

To recap, the pancreas secretes insulin. Insulin is the hormone that enables the uptake of glucose from the blood into bodily tissues. In prediabetes and type 2 diabetes, the cells of the tissues do not generally respond to the action of insulin-this is known as insulin resistance.

To overcome the insulin resistance of the tissues, the pancreas secretes more insulin to try and get the cells to respond and take up glucose from the blood. Eventually, the pancreas can no longer keep up and supply the body with its demand for insulin.

It is this imbalance between supply and demand which leads to raised blood glucose levels. Ultimately, this can lead to exhaustion of the cells of the pancreas that secrete insulin. And this, as mentioned above, is known as B-cell failure.[12]

Type 2 diabetes is commonly found in individuals 45-years of age and older. However, with the advent of processed foods and sedentary lifestyles, more and more young adults, teens, and children are also diagnosed with type 2 diabetes.

As a result, more than 34 million Americans have diabetes, and approximately 90-95% are people with type 2 diabetes. The same diagnostic tests used to diagnose prediabetes are used to diagnose type 2 diabetes. However, the outcomes of the tests are what distinguishes type 2 diabetes from prediabetes.

The table below looks at the different values obtained from diagnostic tests to distinguish between diabetes and prediabetes.

Result	Fasting blood glucose	Random blood glucose	A1C test	Oral glucose tolerance test
Diabetes	>126mg/dL (6.99mmol/L)	> 200mg/dL (11.1mmol/L)	> 6.5%	> 200mg/dL (11.1mmol/L)
Prediabetes	100-125mg/dL (5.55-6.94mmol/L)	N/A	5.7-6.4%	140-199mg/dL (7.77-11.04mmol/L)

Table 2: outcomes of diagnostic tests which distinguish type 2 diabetes from prediabetes.[13]

Because type 2 diabetes is usually preceded by prediabetes (which is often asymptomatic or presents with vague symptoms), symptoms typically develop over a number of years- hence why type 2 diabetes is usually diagnosed in individuals over 45-years of age.

Increased urination, increased thirst, and unintentional loss of weight are very common symptoms of diabetes. Other symptoms include increased hunger, blurred vision, tingling sensations in the hands and feet, increased lethargy, dry skin, delayed healing of wounds, and more infections than usual.[14]

Other risk factors for developing type 2 diabetes include prediabetes and non-alcoholic fatty liver disease.[15]

As with any disease, the ultimate "kicker" is not the cause of the disease, the underlying mechanism of the disease process, or the symptoms but rather the complications of the disease. Type 2 diabetes has a number of possible complications, both acute (sudden onset) and chronic (prolonged and insidious onset).

A common acute complication of type 2 diabetes is hyperglycemic hyperosmolar syndrome, which occurs when blood glucose levels are incredibly high for a prolonged period. When this happens, it becomes a medical emergency.[16]

Chronic complications of type 2 diabetes arise from damaged blood vessels, nerves, and organs due to prolonged high blood glucose levels. Even mildly prolonged elevated blood glucose levels can lead to complications. Therefore, type 2 diabetes has vast complications.

Individuals with type 2 diabetes are five times more likely to develop heart disease or have a stroke. This is because there is an alteration in the body's fat metabolism (as glucose is in the blood and cannot be used by the body's tissues as a source of energy), leading to atherosclerosis (blood vessels become narrowed by fatty substances).

The narrowing of the blood vessels then leads to an alteration in the blood flow (imagine a pipe that becomes slightly blocked), compromising the blood supply to the heart, causing angina (heavy, dull, or tight chest pain). If a blood vessel in the heart or brain becomes completely occluded, this is what results in a heart attack or stroke.[17]

Blood supply to the lower limbs may also become compromised, which leads to peripheral vascular disease- individuals with peripheral vascular disease usually complain of pain in the calves while walking; this is known as claudication.[18]

Another complication is nerve damage which results from damage to the small blood vessels that supply the nerves. Nerve damage can result in a tingling sensation and numbness of the limbs and alteration in the normal gut function resulting in nausea, vomiting, constipation, or diarrhea.

Due to numbness of the feet, people with diabetes do not realize when they have had an injury to their feet. This minor injury can lead to a sizeable ulcerating wound if this goes unchecked- hence why people with diabetes are told to check their feet for cuts and abrasions daily.[19]

People with diabetes are also known to suffer from decreased vision. This is because the blood vessels of the retina (the light-sensitive layer of tissue of the eye) can become occluded, leaky, or grow haphazardly.[20]

Altered kidney function is yet another complication of diabetes. Due to compromised blood supply, the kidneys cannot function optimally, and it is usually associated with high blood pressure. In rare and severe cases, this may also lead to kidney failure.[21]

Another complication of diabetes is sexual dysfunction. For example, men often have erectile dysfunction-especially if they have a significant smoking history. Likewise, a woman may experience loss of libido, vaginal dryness, pain during sex, and may also have less ability to orgasm.[22]

Due to a compromised blood supply to the placenta during pregnancy, pregnant diabetic women have a higher chance of suffering from a miscarriage and birthing a stillborn. In addition, there is also a higher chance of the baby being born with congenital disabilities.[23]

Reading the above complications of type 2 diabetes seems downright depressing, right? Well, the only way to prevent the complications is to manage type 2 diabetes optimally.

There are a variety of medications on the market that can aid in this; however, what if some lifestyle and dietary changes could bring about remission? Think about it, alterations in a person's diet and leading a more active lifestyle can put type 2 diabetes into remission and improve one's general well-being and mood.[24]

Studies have shown that a combination of lifestyle modifications and weight loss (in overweight and obese individuals) can reverse glucose impairment. It must be noted here that a restricted diet is not suitable in persons with reduced kidney or liver function, cardiac impairment, and eating disorders.[25]

Research has proven that there are tremendous benefits to just losing 5% of your body weight. Substantial and suitable **(under medical supervision)** weight loss can lead to taking fewer medications to control your blood glucose levels; it can improve blood glucose levels and lower the risk of developing complications.

In addition, it is thought that weight reduction aids in decreasing the amount of fat that surrounds the pancreas and liver, which leads to improved insulin secretion by the pancreas and improves the glucose metabolism by the liver.

However, it is important to note that the above-mentioned weight loss and lifestyle changes must be maintained to keep type 2 diabetes in remission and always kept under medical supervision.[26]

As we have just discussed, weight loss (in suitable candidates) and lifestyle changes can result in the remission of type 2 diabetes. But what does suitable mean? Body mass index (BMI), as mentioned earlier, is a widely used screening tool used to establish if one is underweight, normal, overweight, or obese, which is calculated by a person's weight (in kg) divided by their square of height (in meters).

The result is interpreted as follows: underweight has a BMI lower than 18.5, normal between 18.5-25, overweight between 25-30, and obese is higher than 30.[27]

However, the tool is slightly flawed. For example, a body builder may have a BMI of 27; however, this does not mean they have excess fat. One may also have a normal BMI but still have a significant amount of fat surrounding their pancreas, liver, and other organs (visceral fat)-this is known as metabolically obese normal weight (MONW).

In instances like this, where a person has been diagnosed with prediabetes or type 2 diabetes, but their BMI is normal, lifestyle and dietary modifications can still aid in type 2 diabetes remission by decreasing the amount of visceral fat. To put it simply, one can be lean but not healthy.[28]

Going back to the DPP study, it showed that through lifestyle changes, it is possible to prevent type 2 diabetes in the background of prediabetes.

There is a significant difference between group 1 (these candidates received intense training on lifestyle changes) who decreased their risk of developing diabetes by 58%, and group 2 (these candidates were given an oral hypoglycemia agent and had only some training on lifestyle changes) who decreased their chances of developing diabetes by 31%.

Traditionally, according to society's dogma, pharmaceutical interventions should have a more significant effect than simple lifestyle changes. This book explores the lifestyle changes shown to put prediabetes and type 2 diabetes into remission. Although certain lifestyle changes may seem challenging at first, they are all relatively simple and logical.

Throughout this book, we will discuss and explore different lifestyle changes, from dietary changes and strategies to the importance of regular exercise and the importance of sleep and water. We will also explore the importance of mental health. And, of course, like any other wellness journey, we will discuss the importance of cessation of smoking.

For one to successfully achieve remission, one has to have a holistically sound approach. In the words of Jan Mundo, "be willing to do whatever it takes to be a warrior for your own health."

2

DIET PART ONE: CULTIVATE A CLEAN AND HEALTHY DIET

In Chapter 1, we defined prediabetes and type 2 diabetes. Then, we discussed how one "gets" prediabetes and type 2 diabetes. We also discussed the DPP (Diabetes Prevention Program) study, and we explored their findings.

In one sentence, we can conclude that to achieve remission and prevent type 2 diabetes, one must change their thoughts and behaviors towards food.

In this chapter, we will look at what it means to cultivate a clean and healthy diet. The aim of cultivating a clean and healthy diet is to help restore normal blood glucose levels.

A diet high in processed foods and red meats are important risk factors for developing prediabetes. Therefore, a diet low in red meats and processed foods are an important factor in preventing and even "reversing" prediabetes and Type 2 diabetes.

Processed foods are high in calories, fats, and sugars-often without any nutritional value.[1]

To put prediabetes into remission and ultimately prevent type 2 diabetes, one must consider (and ultimately incorporate) healthier food choices into one's diet.[2]

This is an age-old tale, and we've all heard it a dozen times over. But what is the basis of this, and why, at every corner, are we constantly being told to "incorporate healthier food choices"? To put it simply, by eating healthier and cleaner foods, one does not send one's pancreas into a state of overdrive.

Fundamentally, eating clean means incorporating more whole foods and limiting one's intake of highly processed foods.[3]

Processed foods refer to implementing procedures or methods that ultimately alter the initial food product from its natural state.[4]

Not all processed foods are equal. The NOVA groups for food processing classifies processed foods into four groups:

- **Group 1-** These are unprocessed or minimally processed foods. Unprocessed foods are edible parts of plants such as seeds and fruits or unprocessed animal products such as eggs. Foods that are minimally processed are natural foods altered by processes to preserve them or make them safe to consume, such as the pasteurization of dairy products.[5]
- **Group 2-** processed culinary ingredients. These are derived from group 1 foods or are derived from nature by a variety of processes. These foods are not meant to be consumed by themselves and are usually used in combination with group 1 foods. Examples of Group 2 processed foods include oil, butter, sugar, and salt.[6]
- **Group 3-** processed foods. These are foods that are edible by themselves and can be used in combination with other foods. Group 3 foods include canned vegetables, cheese, bread, canned fish, and fruits in syrup.[7]
- **Group 4-** ultra-processed foods. These foods are made from formulations. Therefore, they contain little or no intact group 1 foods. Group 4 foods include soft drinks, packaged snacks, reconstituted meat products, and pre-prepared frozen dishes.[8]

Group 4 foods are often more tempting to consume because of their convenience, whereas group 1 and group 2 foods can be tedious and inconvenient to prepare. However, this can be overcome by starting with simple meals such as Greek yogurt with fresh berries for breakfast.[9]

SO, WHAT EXACTLY IS CLEAN EATING, AND MOST IMPORTANTLY, WHERE DOES ONE BEGIN?

Clean eating refers to the consumption of fresh, nutritious, and minimally processed foods. Clean eating also supports sustainable agricultural and environmentally sound food practices.[10]

Think of clean eating as prioritizing group 1 and group 2 processed foods, minimizing one's intake of group 3 processed foods, and avoiding group 4 processed foods.

Now, in order to practice clean eating, one should be familiar with the principles of clean eating:

- The first thing one should do is incorporate fruits and vegetables into one's diet. Fruits are a natural source of sugar, but they should generally be limited to one cup or less per serving.
- Instead of just eating any fruit, opt for lower-sugar-containing fruits like berries and kiwi. In addition, to facilitate a slower rate of glucose

entering the bloodstream; one should pair fruit with a source of protein like a handful of seeds or nuts.[11]

The next chapter will discuss why some fruits are better than others for a prediabetic and type 2 diabetic diet but before then, let us look at what we should be doing and avoiding.

- Avoid highly processed foods and always read food and packaging labels. This seems like a tedious and down-right annoying task. Still, it is essential to ascertain if there are any unwanted preservatives, added sugars, or unhealthy fats in the food product.[12]
- Avoid refined carbohydrates such as breakfast cereals.[13]
- Replace "white foods" (e.g., white rice, white bread, and white pasta) with quinoa, barley, and sweet potatoes.[14]
- Avoid vegetable oils and spreads as they are highly processed and often contain small amounts of artificial trans fats. When cooking in oil, olive oil is a better alternative to other vegetable oils.[15]
- Avoid foods with added sugars such as syrups, candy, desserts, sweets, and baked goods.[16]
- Minimize or eliminate your alcohol intake. Alcoholic beverages are a source of undesired carbohydrates. Instead, choose spirits with no-

calorie mixtures, light beers, spritzers, or dry wines.[17]

- Substitute vegetables in recipes. For example, one can substitute finely chopped cauliflower for rice.[18]
- Avoid pre-packaged snack foods like crackers, granola bars, and muffins as they often contain unhealthy ingredients.[19]
- Prioritize water over other beverages.[20]
- Choose food from ethically raised animals.[21]
- And finally, do not skip meals, as this may lead to overeating later. Eating late at night should also be avoided as it is associated with elevated glucose levels in those with prediabetes.[22]

Now it makes no sense to implement the principles of clean eating into one's diet but not do so in a proportionate manner. Hence, clean eating with a balanced diet goes hand-in-hand.

BUT WHAT EXACTLY IS A BALANCED DIET?

A balanced diet refers to a diet with a proportionate amount of necessary foods for optimal health. It contains essential nutrients with a reasonable ratio of all food groups.[23]

Without a balanced diet, one's body is prone to infection, disease, and fatigue. Therefore, a balanced diet is based on two factors; the "right" foods in a "reasonable" proportion.

First, we will discuss the "right" foods and why they are essential for normal bodily function.

A balanced diet incorporates all five major food groups: fruits, vegetables, grains, dairy, and proteins.[24] These are the "right" foods to eat.

Fruits are high in natural sugars, fiber, vitamins (particularly vitamin C), potassium, and antioxidants.[25] Recommended fresh fruits include apples, blueberries, grapefruit, grapes, peaches, pears, and plums.[26]

Vegetables are high in vitamins C and A, folic acid, potassium, fiber, and antioxidants. In addition, they are naturally low in fat and cholesterol. For a full range of nutrients, one should eat vegetables of different colors. Dark and leafy vegetables such as spinach, kale, and green beans are a rich resource of many nutrients.[27]

Whole grains are recommended over refined white flour as most of the nutrients of grain products are found in its outer shell or in the hull of the grain-this is often removed during manufacturing refined white flour.

Therefore, refined white flour has limited nutritional value, whereas whole grains are packed with magnesium, vitamin B, minerals, and fiber. Therefore, try opting for whole-grain bread, pasta, and rice.[28]

Dairy products are good sources of vitamin D, calcium, vitamin A, potassium, and fats. Vitamin D and calcium are essential for good bone health.

Therefore, one should opt for low-fat dairy products such as low-fat milk and low-fat yogurt as they contain less saturated fats, cholesterol, and calories while still having high nutritional value.[29]

Proteins are essential for wound healing and immune function; they allow for metabolic reactions to take place. Proteins also provide for the body's structural framework, and they are responsible for the transportation and storage of nutrients; proteins are also essential for the body's normal functioning.[30]

When it comes to proteins, there are two primary sources; animal-based proteins and plant-based proteins. Healthy animal-based products include poultry, salmon, and sardines. Bearing in mind that red meats have also been linked to an increased risk of cancer, heart disease, and other diseases.

Plant-based proteins include lentils, beans, peas, almonds, and walnuts.[31] Animal-based proteins are also rich in vitamin B- 12, while legumes are rich in folate. Eggs are also an excellent source of vitamin A.

Now that we have discussed the "right" foods, we will now discuss eating the "right" foods in a "reasonable" proportion.

The USDA's (United States Department of Agriculture) "ChooseMyPlate" initiative recommends filling half of one's plate with fruits and vegetables, filling just over one quarter with grains, just under one quarter with protein-containing foods, and adding dairy or a non-dairy substitute on the side.[32]

Diagram 1: What your plate should look like:

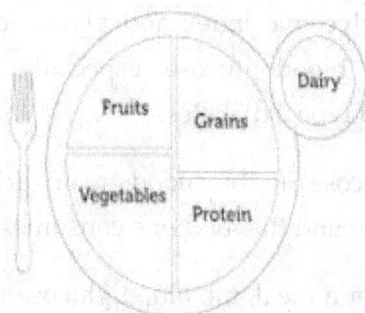

A BALANCED DIET BALANCES THE GLYCEMIC LOAD ON THE BODY (THE GLYCEMIC LOAD WILL BE EXPLAINED FURTHER DOWN). WHAT DOES THIS MEAN?

This means that a meal does not lead to the spiking of blood glucose levels. Instead, there is a lower glycemic response to the meal-hence one does not send one's pancreas into a state of overdrive.

To put this into perspective, a 1-cup serving of peanuts has a glycemic load of 1.6, whereas a 1-cup serving of white rice has a glycemic load of 43. Therefore, the body's glycemic response to a cup of peanuts is less potent than to a cup of white rice.[33]

We shall now discuss this concept in further detail.

Metabolism of carbohydrates is essential in the development of prediabetes and type 2 diabetes. Therefore, to prevent and reverse prediabetes and type 2 diabetes, one needs to understand the metabolism of carbohydrates and how the glycemic index and glycemic load of food products affect blood glucose, especially in those with prediabetes and type 2 diabetes.

Essentially, glucose in the bloodstream arises from two sources: the liver and the food one consumes.[34]

During and after a meal, the blood glucose levels rise. The rise in the level of glucose in the blood signals the pancreas to secrete insulin. As the body cells absorb glucose from the blood (the role of insulin is to encourage glucose uptake from one's blood into the body's cells), the glucose level in the blood begins to fall. When the glucose level in the blood starts to fall, the pancreas then begins to secrete glucagon.

Glucagon, like insulin, is another hormone, which signals the liver to start releasing stored glucose to raise the blood glucose level. The relationship between insulin and glucagon maintains a state of blood glucose equilibrium.[35]

Realistically, the only factor one can control is the quality and quantity of food that one eats, which will determine how quickly or slowly the level of glucose in the blood rises.[36]

In the past, carbohydrates were classified as "simple" or "complex."

WHAT ARE SIMPLE CARBOHYDRATES?

They are fructose and glucose, which have a simple chemical structure composed of only one sugar (monosaccharides) or two sugars (disaccharides).

Due to their simple chemical nature, they are metabolized quickly, leading to a rapid rise in blood glucose and insulin secretion. On the other hand, complex carbohydrates have a more complex chemical nature and consist of three or more sugars (oligosaccharides and polysaccharides).

Due to their more complex chemical nature, they take longer to metabolize and lead to a less immediate and intense impact on the blood glucose level.[37]

However, classifying carbohydrates into simple or complex is simply inadequate. This classification does not account for the effect that carbohydrates have on blood glucose. Also, it does not give an idea of how much digestible carbohydrate the food product contains. Therefore, to help understand this, the glycemic index and glycemic load were developed.[38]

The glycemic index accounts for how different carbohydrate-rich foods directly affect blood glucose levels. It is also a better way of classifying carbohydrates-especially starchy carbohydrates (e.g., white bread).

Starchy carbohydrates are considered complex carbohydrates but are not necessarily the healthiest to eat.[39]

Now, the glycemic index ranks carbohydrates based on how quickly and how much they raise the blood glucose level after eating.

The scale of the glycemic index ranges from 0 to 100. Low-glycemic foods are rated at 55 or less, medium glycemic foods have a rating between 56-69, and high-glycemic foods are rated between 70 to 100.[40]

Foods with a higher glycemic index, like white bread, are quickly digested, which leads to major fluctuations in the blood glucose level. Foods with a lower glycemic index have the opposite effect. They are digested at a slower rate which leads to a gradual rise in blood glucose levels.

Many factors affect a food's glycemic index. These include processing (highly processed foods are more likely to have a higher glycemic index), physical form (whole form grains like brown rice and oats are less rapidly digested than finely ground grain and therefore take longer to digest.), fiber content (high- fiber foods are digested more slowly as they don't contain as many easily digestible carbohydrates compared to low-fiber foods), fat and acid content (fat and acid are digested at a slower rate), and ripeness (ripe fruits and vegetables tend to have a higher glycemic index than unripened fruits and vegetables).[41]

The following are some examples of low, medium, and high glycemic index food products:

- Low-glycemic food products are barley, white spaghetti, raw apple, raw oranges, raw dates, boiled carrots, vegetable soup, full-fat milk, skimmed milk, chickpeas, and lentils.[42]
- Medium-glycemic foods are wheat roti, specialty grain bread, couscous, muesli, mango, raw pineapple, boiled sweet potato, popcorn, and potato chips.[43]
- High-glycemic foods are boiled white rice, rice porridge, instant oat porridge, watermelon, boiled potato, instant mash, rice milk, and rice crackers/chips.[44]

Now, the glycemic load helps establish how different sized portions of different foods compare in terms of their blood glucose-raising effect.[45]

This is because the glycemic load takes into account the amount of carbohydrates in the food product in relation to its impact on the blood glucose level as the glycemic index does.

A food's glycemic load is calculated by multiplying its glycemic index by the amount of carbohydrate in the food product.

A glycemic load that is ten or less is considered a low glycemic load, 11 to 19 is considered a medium glycemic load, and 20 or more is considered a high glycemic load.[46]

Knowing the glycemic load is valuable to those with prediabetes and type 2 diabetes as it aids in assessing which foods are suitable for maintaining normal blood glucose levels.[47]

The following are examples of the low, medium, and high glycemic load food products:

- Examples of low glycemic load food products are bran cereals, apples, oranges, kidney beans, black beans, lentils, skimmed milk, cashews, and peanuts.[48]
- Examples of medium glycemic load food products are ¾ cup of cooked brown rice, 1 cup of cooked oatmeal, three rice cakes, one slice of whole-grain bread, and one ¼ cup of cooked whole-grain pasta.[49]
- Examples of high glycemic load food products are baked potato, French fries, sugar-sweetened beverages, white basmati rice, and white-flour pasta.[50]

There are many schools of thought when it comes to a prediabetic and type 2 diabetic diet. One is following a diet with food products that have a low glycemic index and load. Another approach is following a low-carbohydrate-high-fat diet. Some even advocate for combining the two diets together.

The choice of which diet to follow should be based on personal preference and in conjunction with a medical professional.

In the next chapter, we will discuss the principles of following a low-carbohydrate diet. First, however, it is important to know which carbohydrates to eat and which to avoid. In other words, how to "cut carbs the right way."

3

DIET PART TWO: CUTTING CARBS
THE RIGHT WAY

The previous chapter discussed what clean and healthy eating was and concluded that it comprises two components; opting for wholesome and nutritious foods in good and reasonable proportions.

We also discussed the glycemic index and glycemic load concepts and their significance, especially for those with prediabetes and type 2 diabetes.

In this chapter, we will delve into more depth about carbohydrates and discover that carbohydrates are not only found in starchy foods.

Carbohydrates (carbs) are usually found in starches and sugars. When carbohydrates are digested, they are converted into glucose and absorbed into the bloodstream.

The more carbohydrates are eaten at a meal; the more glucose is absorbed into the bloodstream resulting in a rise in the blood glucose level.[1]

Carbohydrates are the nutrients that significantly raise blood glucose levels and require the most insulin for metabolism.[2]

It seems pretty evident that sugary foods are not suitable for one's health, but what is not so obvious is that some foods, such as fruits, contain a high amount of sugar. Albeit natural sugar, it does not necessarily mean it is a "good carbohydrate"-especially in the background of prediabetes and type 2 diabetes.

Starchy foods (such as bread, rice, pasta, and potato) are loaded with carbohydrates and quickly raise the blood glucose level once digested.[3]

It is vital to note that different carbohydrates will affect individuals differently-this phenomenon is based on genetics and an individual's baseline insulin sensitivity.

For example, eating a potato could raise one person's blood glucose level by as much as eating nine teaspoons of sugar while not affecting another person's blood glucose that intensely.

Hence, by testing one's blood glucose level before eating and then every 30 minutes after eating for up to 2 hours, one can establish which food products cause extreme spikes in one's blood glucose levels and which don't.

Ultimately, one should be able to figure out which food products have the most significant effect on one's blood glucose. And therefore, one can individualize which foods to include and exclude in their diet.[4]

In 2019, the American Diabetes Association published a consensus report that found that individuals with diabetes who reduced their overall carbohydrate intake demonstrated the most evidence for improving blood glucose levels.

The report emphasized that there is no "one-size-fits-all" eating pattern to prevent or manage prediabetes or diabetes.

The report also acknowledged that it is unrealistic to expect that there should be a particular eating pattern for those with prediabetes and diabetes due to different cultural backgrounds, personal preferences, socio-economic backgrounds, and co-occurring conditions.[5]

Another systematic review and meta-analysis of dietary carbohydrate restriction in patients with type 2 diabetes found that low-to-moderate carbohydrate diets have a better effect on glycemic control in type 2 diabetes than high-carbohydrate diets.

It also found that the greater the carbohydrate restriction, the greater the lowering of blood glucose levels.[6]

From analyzing the data from the above two mentioned reports, we can conclude that one is better positioned to control their blood glucose level by restricting one's carbohydrate intake.

A low-carb diet limits carbohydrate intake. It restricts the intake of starchy vegetables, grains, and fruits while encouraging food consumption that is high in protein and "good" fat.

This is called a low-carb-high-fat diet (LCHF) or, in other words, a keto diet, bearing in mind that not all low-carb diets result in ketosis.

Now, those that are taking medication for diabetes (such as insulin) or for hypertension, a woman that is breastfeeding, and those with chronic medical conditions should not immediately start a low-carb-high-fat diet without first consulting a medical professional.[7]

It is important to note that "low-fat" foods are often just simply nothing more than a gimmick.

BUT WHY IS THIS?

Low-fat food products are often loaded with sugar to overcome the low-fat content of the food product.[8]

However, not all low-fat food products are compensated with carbohydrates, which means that one must be carbohydrate-wise when choosing low-fat food products.

Low-carb, high-fat diets stabilize the blood glucose level. This, in turn, causes the level of insulin to drop. Remember, insulin is the primary fat-storing hormone.

Therefore, by reducing insulin levels, fat is utilized as a source of energy for the body. In other words, fat burning is increased, and this, in turn, facilitates weight loss.[9]

In general, a low-carb diet is defined as any diet below 130 grams of carbohydrates per day.[10] However, a low-carb diet does not mean a no-carb diet.[11]

One should opt for fish, eggs, poultry, vegetables that grow above the ground, and natural fats while avoiding sugary and starchy foods like white bread, pasta, potatoes, and white rice.[12]

Table one demonstrates which food products are loaded with carbohydrates and which aren't. Please note that the table is being used as a tool for educational purposes only; it is in no way promoting calorie counting or weighing foods.

Food product	Grams of digestible carbohydrates per 100 grams (3 ½ ounces)
Natural fats (e.g., butter and olive oil)	0
Fish and seafood	0
Meat	0
Eggs	1
Cheese	1
Vegetables that grow above ground	1-5
Fruit	6-20
Potato	15
Beer	13
Cooked rice	28
Cooked pasta	29
Bread	46
Chocolate bar	60

Table 1: food products and their corresponding grams of digestible carbohydrates per 100 grams (3 ½ ounces).[13]

A point to note here is that low-carb-high-fat diets do not require calorie counting or the weighing of foods. Instead, one should eat when one is hungry and stop when one is full.[14] Also, low-fat foods should *always* be avoided.[15]

Fruits are loaded with natural sugars. However, just because these sugars are natural does not mean that they are suitable for a low-carbohydrate diet.[16]

Table two shows the carbohydrate content of some fruits and demonstrates that not all fruits are equal when it comes to carbohydrate content.

Fruit	Portion size	Grams of digestible carbohydrates per portion size
Raspberry	½ a cup (60 grams)	3
Blackberry	½ a cup (70 grams)	4
Strawberry	8 medium-sized (100 grams)	6
Plum	1 medium-sized (65 grams)	7
Clementine	1 medium-sized (75 grams)	8
Kiwi	1 medium-sized (70 grams)	8
Cherry	½ cup or about 12 (75 grams)	8
Blueberry	½ cup (75 grams)	9
Cantaloupe	1 cup (160 grams)	11
Peach	1 medium-sized (150 grams)	13
Orange	1 large-sized	17
Apple	1 medium-sized	21
Banana	1 medium-sized	24

Table 2: fruits and their corresponding grams of digestible carbohydrates per portion size.[17]

As mentioned before, it is unnecessary to count calories or weigh foods before consumption on a low-carb diet but rather be aware of portion size.

Table 2 has been used to explain the types of fruit one should eat and avoid on a low-carb diet. Remember, fruit is not essential in a low-carb diet as all its nutrients can be found in low-carb vegetables instead-without all the added sugar[18].

All this information may seem overwhelming, and one may not know where to begin right now.

But to help you get started, here are some tips:

- **Know what foods are low-carb:** lean meats (sirloin, chicken breast), fish, eggs, green leafy vegetables, cauliflower, broccoli, nuts and seeds, olive oil, some fruits (blueberries and strawberries), whole milk, and Greek yogurt-there are so many more.[19]
- **Choose wisely:** choose foods with a low-carb count but high nutritional value.
- **Make a meal plan:** making a realistic meal plan for one's lifestyle makes it much easier to stick to a low-carb lifestyle.[20]
- **Meal prep:** this helps to avoid unhealthy food choices and saves time and money.
- **Substitution:** use lettuce leaves instead of taco shells, zucchini ribbons instead of pasta, cauliflower pizza crust instead of flour crust, and butternut squash fries instead of traditional ones.[21]
- **Skip** soft drinks and prioritize water.[22]
- **Think ahead when dining out:** choose restaurants whose menu isn't solely based on pasta and bread; instead, opt for seafood restaurants. Also, avoid eating the complimentary bread which is offered.[23]

- **Lose the condiments:** there are lots of carbohydrates hidden in relishes and ketchup.[24]
- **Time for an oil change:** choose olive oil and peanut oil.[25]
- **Cutting the candy:** cut out candy and sweets; instead, opt for a low-carb-containing fruit.

Here are some easy, quick, and delicious recipes to get you going:

Baked chicken in foil with asparagus and garlic lemon butter sauce[26]:

Ingredients:

- Two medium chicken breasts: boneless, skinless, and sliced horizontally.
- Two tablespoons vegetable broth or chicken broth.
- 1 ½ tablespoon of fresh lemon juice.
- Four teaspoons minced garlic (4 cloves).
- Salt and fresh ground black pepper (optional).
- 3-4 tablespoons butter, diced into small cubes.
- Two tablespoons of fresh chopped parsley or cilantro.
- 450g of medium-thick asparagus- trim the woody ends.

Cooking instructions:

- Preheat the oven to 220°C and cut two sheets (35 x 30 cm) of heavy-duty aluminum foil. Lay each piece separately on the countertop. In a small bowl, mix the broth and lemon juice.
- Season the chicken breasts with salt and pepper and divide the chicken onto the aluminum foil near the center. Now place the trimmed asparagus to one side of the chicken, following the long direction of the foil.
- Sprinkle garlic on the chicken breasts and drizzle the sauce generously over the chicken breasts and asparagus.
- Divide the butter pieces evenly among the foil packets. Be sure to layer them over the chicken breasts and asparagus.
- Wrap the chicken foil packets in and crimp the edges together, then wrap the ends up. Don't wrap too tight to keep a little extra space inside for steam to circulate.
- Transfer the chicken foil packs to a baking sheet, bake the chicken in the oven, and continue baking for about 20–25 minutes or until the chicken is cooked.
- Once it's cooked through, remove it from the oven and carefully unwrap the baked chicken in foil packets. If desired, drizzle more lemon juice.

Butter lemon garlic steak and broccoli skillet[27]:

Ingredients:

- 650g of sirloin steak sliced against the grain.
- Two broccoli heads cut into florets.
- Two tablespoons of olive oil.
- Four garlic cloves-minced.
- Three tablespoons of butter (or ghee).
- Juice of half a lemon.
- 60ml of low-sodium beef broth.
- ¼ cup of chopped parsley.
- ¼ teaspoon of crushed red pepper flakes (optional).
- Fresh cracked black pepper.
- Fresh thyme.

The steak marinade: 1/3 cup of low-sodium soy sauce, ½ cup of olive oil, one tablespoon of any hot chili sauce (optional)

Cooking instructions:

- Combine the ingredients for the marinade into a shallow bowl, add the steak strips into the marinade, and allow the steak strips to marinate in the refrigerator for 30 minutes to one hour.
- While waiting for the steak strips to marinate, break down the broccoli heads into florets. Now

blanch the florets into boiling water for 1 or 2 minutes and then rinse with cold water.

- Bring the steak strips to room temperature and heat the olive oil and one tablespoon butter in a large skillet over medium-high heat. Reserve the juices of the marinade for later. Sear the steak strips in batches for 1-2 minutes on each side until the edges are crispy and browned, and add extra olive oil if needed. Now, remove the steak strips from the skillet and set them aside on a plate.
- Using the same skillet, lower the heat to medium. Melt two tablespoons of butter and add the lemon juice, minced garlic, beef broth, and left-over marinade juices. Bring to a simmer. Add the fresh parsley and broccoli florets to the skillet and regularly toss until cooked to your liking.
- Reheat the steak strips quickly by adding them back into the skillet and serve immediately with thyme, chili flakes, more parsley, and lemon slices.

Salmon spinach casserole with cream cheese and mozzarella[28]:

Ingredients:

- Four individual slices of salmon fillets.
- 3.5 grams of softened cream cheese.
- Two cups of rinsed spinach.
- Two tablespoons of olive oil, divided.
- Two grams of shredded mozzarella cheese.
- Three cloves of garlic (minced).
- ½ teaspoon of red pepper flakes (optional).
- ½ teaspoon of Italian seasoning (optional).

Cooking instructions:

- Position a rack in the center of the oven and preheat the oven to 200°C. Add the olive oil, garlic, Italian seasoning, red pepper flakes, one teaspoon of salt, and half a teaspoon of black pepper into a bowl; arrange the salmon fillets in a baking dish and cover them with the marinade. Set the marinated salmon aside for 10-15 minutes on the counter and continue prepping the other ingredients.
- Wilt the spinach in a skillet with one tablespoon olive oil and set aside.
- Spread the softened cream cheese over the salmon fillets and lay the spinach on top of the cream cheese, and sprinkle mozzarella over the top.

- Bake the spinach salmon casserole for 20-25 minutes until the salmon is cooked through. Sprinkle with red chili pepper flakes and chopped parsley, and serve the spinach salmon casserole warm.

Tuscan soup[29]:

Ingredients:

- 450g of hot Italian or turkey sausage with the casings removed.
- One large chopped onion.
- Three cloves of garlic (minced).
- One teaspoon of dried oregano.
- Half a cup of drained and chopped sun-dried tomatoes.
- Salt and freshly ground black pepper.
- Six cups of low-sodium chicken broth.
- One bunch of kale with the leaves stripped and chopped.
- ¾ cup of heavy whipping cream.
- ¼ cup of freshly grated Parmesan.
- And fresh chopped parsley.

Cooking instructions:

- Set a 6-qt Instant Pot to sauté mode. Add the Italian sausages to the insert of the Instant Pot and cook. Break the sausages up with a wooden spoon until the sausages are lightly browned. Now drain the excess fat.
- Add the garlic, onion, and oregano to the Instant Pot. Stir the contents constantly until the onions have become translucent.
- Stir in the chicken broth and sun-dried tomatoes and season with pepper.
- Select the manual setting on the Instant Pot. Adjust the pressure to high and set the timer for 5 minutes. When the sausage soup has finished cooking, do a quick release. Select the sauté mode and stir the kale in the soup until wilted. Stir in the heavy cream until heated through-this takes about 1 minute. Add the salt and pepper and serve immediately with freshly grated Parmesan and parsley.

Creamy cauliflower and broccoli stir-fry with sun-dried tomatoes[30]:

Ingredients:

- One head of broccoli-broken up into small florets.
- Half a head of riced head cauliflower.
- One medium-sized minced onion.
- Half a cup of chopped sun-dried tomatoes.
- One tablespoon of olive oil (or coconut oil).
- One teaspoon of paprika.
- One teaspoon of cumin.
- One teaspoon of Italian seasoning.
- Salt and pepper.
- ¼ cup of vegetable broth.
- One cup of creamy coconut milk.

Cooking instructions:

- Heat a large non-stick or cast-iron skillet over medium heat and heat the oil. Stir-fry the onion until fragrant and translucent.
- Add the chopped sundried tomatoes to the onion and continue stir-frying.
- Add the broccoli florets, riced cauliflower, paprika, Italian seasoning, and cumin to the skillet. Stir regularly for 10 minutes until the veggies are crisp.
- Pour the vegetable broth and coconut milk over the cauliflower and broccoli and stir well to mix. Lower the heat and continue cooking for 5 minutes

until the vegetables are done and the cooking
juices have slightly reduced.
- Add salt and pepper and serve immediately.

Vegan and gluten-free zucchini soup[31]:

Ingredients:

- One tablespoon of canola oil.
- ¼ minced yellow onion.
- One medium-diced zucchini.
- One garlic clove (minced).
- Three tablespoons of tomato sauce.
- Half a teaspoon of Italian seasoning.
- Half a teaspoon of red pepper flakes.
- Half a teaspoon of freshly cracked black pepper.
- One teaspoon of fresh basil (minced).
- One cup of low sodium vegetable stock.

Cooking instructions:

- Heat the oil in a pot or saucepan over medium heat. Add the diced onions and sauté until translucent.
- Add in the diced zucchini and sauté for 1 minute.
- Add the garlic, Italian seasoning, pepper, and red chili pepper flakes. Stir constantly for 1 minute.
- Add and stir in the tomato sauce and minced basil.
- Add the vegetable stock and bring to a simmer. Lower the heat to medium-low. Stir, cover, and cook for about 10 minutes. Make sure to stir once in a while.
- Take the soup off the heat and use a blender until the soup is smooth.
- Divide the soup into bowls. Top the soup with reserved diced zucchini, basil, croutons, and a drizzle of olive oil.

Pan-seared honey balsamic cabbage steaks [32]:

Ingredients:

- One head of green cabbage cut into ¾ -inch-thick slices.
- Four tablespoons of olive oil.
- ¾ teaspoon of coarse salt.
- ½ teaspoon of ground white pepper.
- Two tablespoons of balsamic vinegar.
- Two teaspoons of honey.
- One sprig of fresh thyme.

Cooking instructions:

- Preheat a large skillet over medium heat.
- Combine three tablespoons of olive oil, balsamic vinegar, and honey in a small bowl. Arrange the cabbage slices on a shallow plate and brush them with the honey-balsamic vinaigrette. Add salt and ground pepper and sprinkle with thyme.
- Add one tablespoon of olive oil to the skillet. Transfer the cabbage steaks to the hot skillet. Cook on both sides until cabbage slices are crisp-tender and the edges are golden. Brush the cabbage steaks regularly with the honey-balsamic mixture.
- Serve immediately. Add salt and pepper to your liking.

Lemon garlic butter zucchini noodles[33]:

Ingredients:

- Four medium-sized zucchinis.
- 3-4 cloves of garlic (minced).
- One cup of fresh chopped cilantro.
- Two tablespoons of butter.
- Juice of half a lemon.
- Half a teaspoon of red crushed chili pepper flakes (optional).
- One tablespoon of hot sauce of your choice.

Cooking instructions:

- Trim, wash, and pat dry the ends of the zucchini. Next, make the noodles using a spiralizer or a julienne peeler.
- In a large skillet, over medium heat, melt two tablespoons of butter. Add the lemon juice, hot sauce, minced garlic, half the cilantro, and the red pepper flakes.
- Add the zucchini noodles and cook them for 3 or 4 minutes. Make sure to stir regularly and coat the noodles in the butter sauce until the zucchini is done but still crisp. Add salt and pepper and garnish with remaining fresh cilantro. Serve immediately.

Brown butter garlic cauliflower foil pockets[34]:

Ingredients:

- One cauliflower head-broken down into florets and rinsed.
- Five cloves of grated garlic.
- 1 or 2 teaspoons of dried garlic (optional).
- 1 or 2 teaspoons of dried oregano.
- Salt and freshly cracked pepper.
- 1/3 cup of brown butter (or ghee).
- Fresh chopped parsley.
- Fresh thyme leaves.
- Crushed red chili pepper flakes (optional).

Cooking instructions:

- Preheat the oven to 200°C.
- Cut four sheets of foil (about 40cm long). Divide the cauliflower florets into four equal portions and arrange them in the center of each foil sheet.
- Slightly fold the sides up of each foil sheet. Add the grated garlic, oregano, thyme, salt, and pepper. Pour the browned butter over the cauliflower and gently toss. Fold the sides of the foil sheets over the cauliflower florets, ensuring that they are completely closed and sealed.
- Place the foil pockets on a rimmed baking sheet and bake until cooked through. This should take about 15- 20 minutes.

- Serve immediately. Add the red crushed chili pepper flakes, fresh parsley, fresh thyme, and more brown butter.

In Chapter 4, we will discuss intermittent fasting and how, on a physiological level, intermittent fasting can help in aiding in achieving remission from prediabetes and type 2 diabetes.

4

FASTING IS YOUR FRIEND: A QUICK GUIDE TO INTERMITTENT FASTING

We have now discussed clean and healthy eating, the importance of the glycemic index and glycemic load in a prediabetic and diabetic diet, and how to cut carbs the right way. Combining all this knowledge, this chapter will discuss what intermittent fasting is and some of the approaches to intermittent fasting.

Although intermittent fasting has gained popularity over the past few years, it is in no way a "new" diet fad. Our forefathers have been practicing intermittent fasting for centuries-mainly for religious and spiritual reasons.

For example, Ramadhan is observed in the Islamic faith whereby its followers fast for 29 or 30 days and abstain from eating and drinking from dawn to sunset.

The Daniel Fast is observed by some Christians and is a partial fast rather than a restricted fast and is usually observed for 21 days.

Those who practice Judaism fast for 24 hours on seven significant days of their religious year.

Buddhists also practice fasting. And fasting is also observed in the Hindu faith and is practiced in many forms.

As previously discussed, type 2 diabetes is a disease of insulin resistance. The majority, but not all, of the available medical therapies, aim to provide the body with more insulin. Some medical therapies aim at reducing glucose produced by the liver. It seems somewhat ironic that insulin resistance is treated conventionally by, in essence, "adding" more insulin.

One cannot deny that these conventional medical therapies do aid in preventing hyperglycemia, but they do not address the underlying cause of insulin resistance. Furthermore, it has been demonstrated that using insulin to treat insulin resistance over time can increase a person's medications.[1]

This is where intermittent fasting plays a vital role in the treatment and possible remission of prediabetes and type 2 diabetes. In short, intermittent fasting improves one's insulin sensitivity.[2]

A 2018 study published in the British Medical Journal demonstrated that intermittent fasting is an effective way of managing prediabetes and type 2 diabetes.

By practicing three 24-hour fasting periods per week, all of the candidates that participated in the study were able to completely stop their insulin therapy within three weeks of commencing.

The candidates managed to reduce their HbA1C levels, and two-thirds of them were also able to stop taking all of their type 2 medications. All the candidates also managed to either reduce or completely reverse their insulin resistance, and they also lost a significant amount of weight.[3]

With this being said, it is not wise to completely stop or reduce any medications without first consulting a medical professional.

Broadly speaking, intermittent fasting is based on the principle of consuming very little to no calories for periods that range from 12 hours to several days with a regular pattern. We will discuss several regimes shortly.[4]

Intermittent fasting is also known as therapeutic fasting. In essence, it is an eating program that involves scheduled periods with no food intake. However, one is allowed to consume unlimited amounts of very-low-caloric drinks such as water, coffee, tea, and bone broth.[5]

THERE ARE THREE MAIN INTERMITTENT FASTING PROGRAMS FOR ONE TO CONSIDER:

1. **The 5: 2 plan.** This involves eating "normally" for five days and partially fasting for the other two days of the week.[6]

2. **The 24-hour plan.** This involves eating no food for one to three days of the week. For example, one can eat "normally" the whole of Monday and consider dinner as one's last meal on Monday, and then the next meal will be on Tuesday at dinner time.[7] One thing to note here is that one is not supposed to fast longer than 24 hours. The reason for this will also be discussed shortly.

3. **The time-restricted plan.** This involves dividing the day into two blocks. The idea is that one consumes all of their required calories within an 8–12-hour block and fasts for the remaining 12-16 hours of the day.[8]

In the 5:2 plan eating "normally" refers to following a clean, healthy, and low-carbohydrate diet plan. This involves avoiding simple and refined carbohydrates and prioritizing vegetables, low-sugar-containing fruits, lean proteins, and healthy fats.[9]

Basically, eating "normally" refers to chapters 2 and 3 of this book. With each of the programs, one can drink a limitless amount of low-or-no-calorie beverages.[10]

For intermittent fasting to have the greatest effect, one should avoid snacking at night and between meals- remember; intermittent fasting aims to reduce insulin levels and use fat as the body's primary source of energy.

BUT HOW DOES INTERMITTENT FASTING AID IN WEIGHT LOSS?

Well, food that is consumed undergoes digestion in the gut and ultimately ends up as molecules in the bloodstream. Carbohydrates, particularly simple carbohydrates, are rapidly broken down into sugar, which the body's cells use for energy.

If the body does not "spend" this energy source, it gets stored in fat cells with the aid of insulin. Fat cells are, therefore, a source of "potential energy."

The principle of intermittent fasting is based on the fact that if the body does not receive an immediate energy source, insulin levels will decrease. The body will then use its stored potential energy, which is found in fat, for an immediate energy source.

During this time, fat cells release free fatty acids and glycerol. Hence, fat is "burned off." However, for this to be facilitated, insulin levels must decrease enough and for a long enough time.[11]

It must be noted here that the body is always in need of energy to fulfill its basic functions. However, it must also be noted that different activities require different amounts of energy. For example, less energy is needed by the body when one is sleeping compared to when one is running a marathon.

It has been shown that night-time eating is associated with a higher risk of obesity and diabetes. This is thought to be due to the human body's circadian rhythm-meaning the body has adapted to eating during the daytime and sleeping at night.

The nature of intermittent fasting itself is based on the circadian rhythm-eat during the day and fast overnight.

A study conducted by the University of Alabama, which looked at a small group of obese men with prediabetes, found that intermittent fasting resulted in lower insulin levels and improved insulin sensitivity, and a significant decrease in appetite and even though the participants had restricted eating times, they were not hungry.[12]

The 5:2 intermittent fasting diet has become popular in recent years.

HOW DOES IT WORK?

Well, for five days of the week, one eats the daily calorie requirements advised for people of a healthy weight. For men, this equates to 2500kcal per day, and for women, 2000kcal per day. For the other two days of the week, one only eats 25% of the values mentioned above; men 625kcal per day and women 500kcal per day. Also, note here that the two fasting days can be done on any day of the week but not on two consecutive days.[13]

The 5:2 meal plan differs from person to person and should suit one's needs and lifestyle. Therefore, one should opt for a meal schedule that also suits one's needs and lifestyle.

Choosing a suitable fast day meal schedule may initially result in a lot of trial and error. There is no "cookie-cutter" plan, but one can try eating a small breakfast and an early dinner while skipping lunch altogether or only eating one meal for the day.

If the aforementioned is not suitable, one can also eat three small meals for breakfast, lunch, and dinner.[14]

Due to the fact that calories are so drastically restricted on fast days, it is vital that one chooses one's fasting foods carefully, ensuring that they are rich in nutrients like vegetables which are a great option.

Vegetables are lower in calories compared to animal proteins. Therefore, one can "bulk-up" one's plate. Dark and leafy green vegetables are an excellent way to do this. One should also prioritize small portions of lean proteins such as white fish, lean animal cuts, eggs, peas, lentils, and tofu.

Proteins also aid in keeping one full on fast days. If one has a sweet tooth, one should include low-carbohydrate fruits like strawberries and blackberries-refer back to chapter three to recap on which fruits to avoid and which to include.

Soup is also an excellent option for fasting days, and plain, unsweetened coffee and tea are also acceptable on fast days. Water can be consumed in unlimited amounts. And as discussed throughout this book, refined carbohydrates and processed foods should always be avoided.[15]

The second approach to intermittent fasting is the 24-hour plan. It is also known as the eat-stop-eat approach. You may be thinking that fasting for 24-hours seems rather intense and what is the basis of fasting for a total of 24-hours?

Well, during the first 8 hours of the fast, the body continues to digest the last meal that was consumed. The body is unaware that it will not be getting energy from food within the next 24- hours and therefore continues to use stored glucose as an energy source as it would on any other typical day.

However, after 8 hours of not eating, the body will begin to use fat as its energy source and continue to use fat until the 24-hour fast is over.

The key to remember here is that after 24-hours of fasting, the body will no longer use fat as its energy source. Instead, the body will begin to use proteins as its energy source. Remember that proteins play an integral role in maintaining a variety of structural and metabolic functions. It is for this reason why fasting beyond 24 hours is an absolute no-no.[16]

Some may consider the 24-hour fast more convenient than other types of intermittent fasting. For example, if one chooses to eat their last meal at supper time, the next time one consumes food will be the next day at supper time. Therefore, choosing to fast from supper to supper may be more convenient as most families sit down together at that time.

However, if one has to take medications in the morning, the 24- hour fast may be better done from breakfast to breakfast.

Most recommend that the 24-hour fasting model is carried out three to four times per week but bear in mind that fasting more than twice a week can also increase one's risk for developing heart arrhythmias and hypoglycemia in certain patients.

Fasting is also not advised in pregnant or breastfeeding patients, those with type 1 diabetes, those with eating disorders, and those recovering from surgery.[17]

One may begin the 24-hour fast at any time of day that one chooses. However, it is best to plan one's fast ahead as eating healthy, and nutrient-rich foods will help the body get through the 24-hour fasting period.

Foods with a high fiber content help one feel fuller for longer after eating, while fruits and vegetables due to having high water content will help the body stay hydrated. Before one starts a 24-hour fast, one should try and eat foods rich in protein like beans, whole-grain starches, and dairy products.[18]

During a 24-hour fast, one is allowed to consume calorie-free beverages such as unsweetened coffee, tea, and water. A fair amount of water that the body requires comes from foods. Seeing that during a 24-hour fast, no food is to be consumed, one must drink plenty of water.

There is no set amount of how much water one should drink as the amount of water required differs from person to person and is primarily determined by one's level of physical activity. One should also note that they should only drink water when they are thirsty.[19]

Water also constitutes 55-60% of the body and gives fuel to the body-bear in mind that dehydration of just 2% can result in energy loss of up to 20%.

Water is also necessary for the optimal functioning of organs. It also aids in the transportation of nutrients and waste products and detoxifying heavy metals, nicotine, pesticides, and alcohol.[20] The moral of this is that one must ensure that one's water intake is sufficient to aid in these functions.

After the fast is over, one should continue to eat healthy foods.[21] It is somewhat contradictory to observe a 24-hour fast only to eat highly processed and unhealthy foods once the fast is over. One might consider having a small snack or a light meal to break the fast to prevent oneself from overeating.

The energy deficit that fasting creates facilitates weight loss. Fasting may also reduce one's blood sugar. With this being said, fasting is not intended to induce hypoglycemia. Fasting has also been shown to decrease LDL cholesterol, which is considered the "bad" cholesterol, and reduces inflammation.[22]

It is also important to note that eating only one meal a day may cause dizziness, nausea, irritability, constipation, and low energy levels for some people.[23] If this does occur, one can try two of the other approaches to intermittent fasting.

In addition, due to the body's physiological response to 24-hour fasting, one may experience extreme hunger.[24] But, again, this may be overcome by trying one of the other two approaches to intermittent fasting.

Time-restricted fasting is another approach to intermittent fasting. This eating program refers to only eating during a limited period of the day. The idea is that one should consume all of their calories within an 8–12-hour period and fast for the remaining 12-16 hours.[25]

For instance, one can choose to eat between 10 am-6 pm, and fast from 6 pm-10 am the following day.[26] However, one should select a time-restricted eating program that is suitable for one's lifestyle.

Time-restricted eating is not a "one-size-fits-all" type of eating program. This eating program should be followed daily.

Again, it must be stressed that during the "eating" period, one must make sure to eat healthy and nutritious foods.

Time-restricted eating may aid in weight loss, decrease LDL "bad" cholesterol, increase HDL "good cholesterol," and reduce blood sugar.[27] However, this is dependent on the quality of food that one eats.

Generally speaking, time-restricted eating focuses on when to eat rather than on what to eat.[28] Therefore, for optimal results, one should combine time-restricted eating with a low- carbohydrate diet.

So far, we have discussed different dietary strategies that have been shown to aid in treating prediabetes and type 2 diabetes. When done correctly, these strategies can also help achieve remission.

Although we have discussed diet in detail, we have not yet put much emphasis on weight loss. Therefore, the next chapter is dedicated solely to weight loss and the importance of weight loss in order to achieve remission or at the very least reduce the number of medications required to control type 2 diabetes effectively.

5

LOSING WEIGHT (YOU'RE ALREADY ON YOUR WAY!)

Throughout chapters 2-4, we discussed many approaches to diet when it comes to the remission of prediabetes and type 2 diabetes.

We hinted at and slightly glazed over the topic of losing weight. We even brought forward evidence that shows that excess fat in the liver and pancreas is a contributing factor to prediabetes and type 2 diabetes.

We also discussed the concept of MONW- metabolically obese normal weight. However, the majority of evidence has shown that reducing the fat content of the liver and pancreas is one of the primary keys to putting prediabetes and type 2 diabetes into remission. Hence, we have dedicated this chapter to weight loss.

Dr. Roy Taylor, Professor of Medicine at the University of Newcastle in the U.K, and his team have shown that sufficient weight loss can put diabetes into remission. Their DiRECT trial (Diabetes Remission Clinical Trial) found that 46% of their participants following a strict liquid diet program were able to achieve remission.

Only 4% of the comparison group that wasn't following a rigorous liquid diet program were also able to achieve remission. The DiRECT trial defined remission as having an HbA1C below 6.5% and discontinuing all diabetes medications for at least two months.[1]

Now, we are not saying that one should follow a strict liquid diet to put one's diabetes into remission. We are just simply stating the conditions that were applied to the trial.

The study involved 306 individuals diagnosed with type 2 diabetes. All of the participants were aged between 20-65 years and had been diagnosed with diabetes within the past six years; they all had a BMI of 27-45kg/m2 and were not receiving insulin.

The study group of participants was put onto a strict liquid diet program which totaled no more than 853 calories per day. They also stopped taking their diabetes and anti-hypertensive medications.

The rigorous liquid diet program lasted for 3-5 months. This was followed by gradual food reintroduction, which lasted 2-8 weeks. They also continued to follow the standard diabetes care guidelines.

It must be noted here that during the liquid diet phase of the trial, participants were told not to exercise as exercising on a low-calorie restricted diet in obese individuals may lead to overeating- clearly; the researchers did not want to take any chances while gathering data in the liquid diet phase! However, during the weight maintenance phase of the program, exercise was encouraged in order to prevent excessive weight gain.[2]

The average baseline weight of the participants was 101kg. The initial results were as follows:

Weight loss	% Who achieved remission
Gained weight during the study	0
0-5 kg (0-11 lbs.)	7
5-10 kg (11-22 lbs.)	34
10-15 kg (22-33 lbs.)	57
>15 kg (33 lbs.)	86

On further analysis of the data, the research team concluded that sufficient and substantial weight loss facilitated better pancreatic B-cell functioning (B-cells are responsible for synthesizing and secreting insulin).

In addition, they found that better B-cell functioning was associated with a reduction in both liver and pancreatic fat. It was also noted that those diagnosed with type 2 diabetes for a brief time were more likely than those diagnosed with type 2 diabetes for many years to achieve remission by weight loss.

This could be because those with long-standing type 2 diabetes had greater liver and pancreatic fat-induced injury. However, even though those with long-standing diabetes had a slimmer chance of achieving remission, it was noted that weight loss might aid in preventing other serious complications associated with type 2 diabetes.[3]

Dr. Taylor also suggested that achieving weight loss of just 10- 15% of a person's body weight may, in fact, result in better B- cell functioning. He postulated that excessive liver and pancreatic fat might induce "dormancy" of pancreatic B-cells.

With this being said, he also acknowledged that there may be a "personal fat threshold" and that, therefore, one individual might have to lose more weight than the person sitting next to them in order to achieve remission.[4]

Weight loss for remission is not only limited to individuals that are obese. We have previously discussed the concept of MONW (metabolically obese normal weight). The DiRECT study found an interdependent relationship between type 2 diabetes and excessive liver and pancreatic fat.

Therefore, one can have a conventionally "healthy weight" and yet have excess liver and pancreatic fat-in other words, be "metabolically obese." This further proves Dr. Taylor's statement that there may be "personal fat thresholds." Broadly speaking, a person with a conventionally normal BMI cannot be expected to lose as much weight as a person who is conventionally obese.[5]

The study also showed that one's likelihood of remission from diabetes is more likely in the first five years after being diagnosed. If one has long-standing diabetes, it does not mean that they will not achieve remission at all. It just means that it is less likely but is still worth giving it a shot.

It has been reported that a patient who had been diagnosed with type 2 diabetes for over 20 years was able to achieve remission through calorie restriction. However, the study also demonstrated that some study participants could not achieve remission even though they had a relatively new diagnosis of type 2 diabetes. However, with the above research results showing a 46% remission rate, losing weight is definitely worth the shot.[6]

From the above, we can infer that to prevent type 2 diabetes (and "control" prediabetes), one should avoid excessive weight gain.

It must be further noted that one should try and maintain weight loss. A follow-up review of the study found that some participants had gained around 2kg but were still in remission-it is fair to say that a 2kg weight gain is in no way excessive.

The fact that these participants maintained a state of remission might have something to do with the "personal fat threshold" that was mentioned earlier.[7]

In another study, scientists from Johns Hopkins University in the U.S.A concluded that those with prediabetes dramatically reduced their chance of developing type 2 diabetes within the next three years if they lost about 10% of their body weight within six months of being diagnosed with prediabetes.

They made this conclusion based on analyzing the Diabetes Prevention Program's (DPP) findings-this study was discussed at length in Chapter 1. To recap the DPP study, more than 3,000 participants were recruited and studied over three years.

The participants were all overweight and hyperglycemic. They were then divided into three groups. The first group received intensive lifestyle intervention training, the second group received some lifestyle intervention training and were given metformin (a drug used to treat hyperglycemia). And the third group received only a placebo.

Overall, the scientists found that those participants who lost only 10% of their body weight (in the intensive lifestyle intervention training group) had an 85% reduced risk of developing type 2 diabetes within the next three years.[8]

When it comes to weight loss, there are a variety of dietary strategies that are available. However, what is just as important as losing weight is maintaining the weight loss. Exercise plays a major role in maintaining weight loss which will be discussed at length in the next chapter.

Before going further into this chapter, let us recap what we have learned so far.

In chapter 2, we discussed cultivating a clean and healthy diet. In essence, one should avoid highly processed foods and refined carbohydrates and instead opt for whole foods, fruits, and vegetables and replace "unnatural" sugars with "natural" sugars.

We also discussed how vital portion size is and discussed the "ChooseMyPlate" initiative, which recommended filling half of one's plate with fruits and vegetables, filling just over one quarter with grains, filling just under one quarter with protein-containing foods, and adding dairy or a non-dairy substitute on the side.[9]

We also discussed simple and complex carbohydrates. Simple carbohydrates are metabolized quickly and lead to a rapid rise in blood glucose levels. In contrast, complex carbohydrates are metabolized at a slower rate than simple carbohydrates, leading to a less rapid rise in blood glucose.

We also discussed that classifying carbohydrates as simple and complex does not account for the effect of carbohydrates on blood glucose and chronic disease and also does not account for how much digestible carbohydrate the food product contains. Hence, the glycemic index and glycemic load were developed. Finally, we concluded by saying that one should prioritize foods with a low glycemic index and glycemic load.[10]

In chapter 3, we discussed "cutting carbs the right way." We concluded that low-carbohydrate-high-fat diets aid in stabilizing blood glucose levels. The importance of this diet is that it facilitates a reduction in insulin levels-remember that insulin is the primary fat-storing hormone.

With a drop in insulin levels, fat is used by the body for energy. Hence, a decrease in insulin leads to the "burning of fat," which results in weight loss. We also stressed that a "low-carb diet" does not mean a "no-carb diet." In fact, a low-carb diet simply refers to any diet which contains less than 130g of carbohydrates per day.

We also looked at different food products and their corresponding amounts of carbohydrates. We concluded that "white foods" contained more digestible carbohydrates than whole foods, and we discovered that not all fruits are equal in their carbohydrate content.[11]

In chapter 4, we discussed the three primary intermittent fasting modalities. First, we explored the principles of intermittent fasting, which is based on the fact that if the body does not receive an immediate energy source, insulin levels will decrease. The body will then use its stored potential energy, which is found in fat, for an immediate energy source.

Then we noted that fasting should not be prolonged by more than 24 hours as after starving for more than 24 hours, proteins will be used as a source of energy rather than fat. Finally, we noted that, traditionally, intermittent fasting could be done at any time of day depending on one's lifestyle.[12]

With all of the above being said, for those with prediabetes and type 2 diabetes, one must always be conscious of the circadian rhythm.

For example, we have previously discussed that nighttime eating is associated with a higher risk of developing diabetes and obesity-this is in part due to the circadian rhythm.

BUT WHAT IS THE CIRCADIAN RHYTHM?

The circadian rhythm simply refers to the body's adaptation to eating during the day and sleeping at night. Hence, one should not eat or snack a few hours before bedtime.[13]

Remember, there is no "one-size-fits-all" approach to losing weight. The weight loss plan (and ultimately weight loss maintenance) is dependent on multiple factors, including one's lifestyle, physical activity level, religious beliefs, personal beliefs, and demographic and geographical location.

So far in this book, we have discussed some effective approaches to weight loss but not all of them. Below are a variety of other approaches which can also aid in weight loss.

Plant-based diets: vegetarianism and veganism have now become popular approaches to plant-based diets, and animal products are restricted for environmental, health, and ethical reasons.

A flexitarian approach also exists, which does allow for animal products in moderation. Now, vegetarianism involves eliminating all meat, poultry, and fish. On the other hand, veganism is the same as vegetarianism, but it also eliminates animal-derived products like gelatin, eggs, honey, and casein. Instead, this diet focuses on eating fruits, vegetables, and whole-grain food products. Plant-based diets aid in weight loss as they are low in calories and high in fiber, and fiber helps one feel fuller for longer. However, plant-based diets are deficient in vitamin B12, vitamin D, calcium, zinc, and omega-3 fatty acids.[14]

The Paleo diet: this diet is based on the foods that were eaten during the Paleolithic era (2.5 million-10 000 years ago). The diet includes lean meats, fruits, vegetables, nuts, and seeds. It also advises against dairy products, legumes, and grains.

This diet is based on the discordance hypothesis-basically, this means that the human body is genetically mismatched to the modern diet. Some studies have shown that the Paleo diet facilitates more weight loss than other diets, improves glucose tolerance, improves blood pressure control, and better appetite management. However, the diet is absent in whole grains and legumes, which are good sources of fiber, vitamins, and nutrients.[15]

Low-fat diets: low-fat diets involve restricting one's daily fat intake to 30% of the daily recommended calories. There are also ultra-low-fat diets that limit one's fat intake to less than 10% of one's total daily calories.

It is advised that those with prediabetes and type 2 diabetes reduce the number of saturated fats in their diet. Saturated fats are often referred to as "bad fats." Saturated fats are usually found in highly processed and unhealthy foods such as potato chips, fatty and processed meats, cheese, butter, and desserts. On the other hand, unsaturated fats are referred to as "good fats." They are found in food products like oily fish, nuts, and avocado.

Fats directly affect cholesterol levels. LDL (low-density lipoprotein) and HDL (high-density lipoprotein) are the two different types of cholesterols. They are both needed by the body for normal physiological functioning. However, high levels of LDL and low levels of HDL are associated with higher risks of heart disease. and it is for this reason, LDL is termed as "bad cholesterol," and HDL is termed as "good cholesterol."

In addition, saturated fats raise LDL and HDL cholesterol and triglycerides (triglycerides are a form of fat in the blood. Higher triglycerides are also associated with higher risks of heart disease).

Conversely, unsaturated fats help to increase HDL levels. In part, HDL is known as "good cholesterol" as it helps eradicate other forms of cholesterol from the body. HDL also helps remove LDL from healed artery walls;

therefore, high levels of HDL help decrease the risk of heart disease.

Low-fat diets have come under fire recently as they often require a relatively high level of carbohydrate intake to overcome the calorie deficit that low-fat diets provide-fats provide twice the number of calories per gram than proteins and carbohydrates.

Low-fat diets have also been criticized as fats that are rich in vitamins A and D. Studies have shown that low-fat diets have been just as effective as low-carb diets for weight loss; However, it seems that low-carb diets are more effective for weight loss in day-to-day living.

Something to note here is that fats are needed for hormone production, nutrient absorption, and overall cell health. Therefore, restricting too much fat can lead to hormonal and nutrient deficiencies. In addition, very low-fat diets have been linked to a higher risk of metabolic syndrome. If one opts to follow a low-fat diet, one must include some unsaturated fats while completely excluding saturated fats.[16]

The Mediterranean diet: this diet embraces foods eaten by countries surrounding the Mediterranean Sea. It is both nutritious and full of flavor. The diet has been linked to lower cancer risks, diabetes, heart disease, and other chronic conditions. This diet advocates eating fruits, vegetables, nuts, seeds, seafood, and extra virgin olive oil. Eggs, poultry, and dairy products are to be eaten in moderation, while red meats are limited.

It also restricts refined grains, trans fats, refined oils, processed meats, added sugar, and highly processed foods in general. The diet is high in antioxidant-rich foods, which help reduce inflammation and oxidative stress by neutralizing free radicals.

The Mediterranean diet is not strictly only a weight loss diet but more of a lifestyle. Unless calories are restricted on the Mediterranean diet, one may not lose weight. The diet can also be costly and may fall short on nutrients.[17]

Weight Watchers (WW): The weight watchers' diet is one of the most popular weight loss programs worldwide. WW is a point-based system that assigns different food products and beverages with a value dependent on their calorie, fat, and fiber contents. For example, a 230-calorie glazed donut is worth 10 points, while 230 calories of yogurt with blueberries and granola is worth only 2 points. To achieve their target weight, one must eat within their set daily points based on one's height, weight, gender, and weight-loss goal.

A review of 45 studies found that those who followed a WW diet lost 2.6% more weight than those who received standard counseling, and that is because WW also offers to counsel its members. Perhaps this is why their members have been more successful at maintaining weight loss after several years. WW is flexible and "user-friendly." However, it may be costly, and its flexibility can be a downfall if its users choose unhealthy foods.[18]

The DASH diet: Dietary Approaches to Stop Hypertension (DASH) is an eating program initially designed to help prevent and treat high blood pressure (hypertension). However, an analysis of 13 studies found that those following the DASH diet lost significantly more weight over 8-24 weeks compared to those following a controlled diet.

The DASH diet emphasizes eating a variety of healthy foods in order to get the correct nutrients. The DASH diet also acknowledges the importance of portion size. It also promotes eating less salt and salt-containing foods and promotes food products like whole grains, low-fat dairy products, and fruits and vegetables. It also encourages limiting alcohol intake to two drinks or less per day for men and one or less per day for a woman.

The DASH diet also doesn't address caffeine consumption and has been shown to reduce blood pressure and several risk factors for heart disease. It may also aid in preventing recurrent depressive bouts and lower the risk of developing breast and colorectal cancer. However, eating too little salt has been linked to increased insulin resistance and increased risk of death in heart failure patients.[19]

The bottom line is that any healthy and nutritious calorie-restricted diet can help one lose weight. One should follow a diet that one is comfortable with. The foods should be flavorful and easy to incorporate into one's lifestyle, which should be satisfying.

The next chapter will discuss and explore why exercise is vital for those with prediabetes and type 2 diabetes.

Healthy eating and exercise go hand in hand. We will discuss aerobic and anaerobic exercise and the importance of combining the two types of exercise forms. We will also examine why exercise is important and explore the biochemistry of exercise on the body in controlling and potentially achieving remission from prediabetes and type 2 diabetes.

6

THE POWER OF REGULAR EXERCISE (AND HOW YOU CAN MAKE IT A HABIT)

I n Chapter 5, we discussed, in detail, why losing weight is essential in those with prediabetes and type 2 diabetes. We discovered that excess fat in the liver and pancreas might be the underlying cause of type 2 diabetes. Therefore, losing weight may aid in the remission of prediabetes and type 2 diabetes.

We also explored various diet options and concluded that there is no "one diet that fits all." We recapped and rediscussed the glycemic index and glycemic load principles, the importance of "cutting carbs" the right way, and the different approaches to intermittent fasting.

We also discussed the advantages and disadvantages of different dietary lifestyles, including vegetarianism and veganism, the Paleo diet, low-fat diets, the

Mediterranean diet, Weight Watchers, and the DASH diet.

Ultimately, we concluded that one with prediabetes or type 2 diabetes must have an effective dietary strategy. One's dietary strategy must be reasonable in portions and nutritious in order to decrease the fat content in the liver and pancreas, as this has shown to be vital in putting prediabetes and type 2 diabetes into remission.

This chapter will now look at the power and importance of regular exercise and how you can make it into a habit that's rewarding.

Kenneth H. Cooper said, "The reason I exercise is for the quality of life I enjoy." Kenneth H. Cooper is a world-renowned medical doctor who has dedicated his life's work to, well, basically, the positive effects that exercise has on the human body.

To sum up all of his work, one must look at the Cooper philosophy: "It is easier to maintain good health through proper exercise, diet, and emotional balance than to regain it once it is lost".[1] Therefore, throughout this chapter, we urge one to keep the Cooper philosophy in mind.

In general, exercise has been shown to help control weight, lower blood pressure, lower the levels of LDL (low-density lipoprotein), which is known as "bad cholesterol," increase the levels of HDL (high-density lipoprotein), which is known as "good cholesterol," strengthen the muscles and bones and reduce anxiety.

In addition, in those with diabetes, it has been shown that regular physical exercise can also lower blood glucose levels and increase the body's sensitivity to insulin, therefore countering insulin resistance.[2]

The theory behind exercise helping to achieve remission from prediabetes and type 2 diabetes is that firstly, excess fat in the liver blunts the liver's response to insulin. This results in increased glucose production and release from the liver.

Secondly, excess fat in the pancreas causes stress on the pancreatic B-cells (which are responsible for insulin secretion). This fat-induced metabolic stress on the pancreatic B-cells causes the B-cells to enter a state of dormancy, meaning they cannot function optimally. Therefore, the pancreas is unable to secrete enough insulin effectively.[3]

As previously discussed in Chapter 5, weight loss aims to restore normal functioning of the liver and pancreas. In this instance, exercise along with a healthy diet helps aid in decreasing the fat content of the liver and the pancreas. Hence, exercise and diet go hand-in-hand.

Thirdly, regular exercise improves the body's sensitivity to insulin. When muscles are active, which occurs during physical activity and exercise, they use glucose as their primary energy source. The use of glucose as a source of energy prevents the accumulation of glucose in the blood, and instead of glucose staying in the blood, glucose is taken up by the muscles.[4]

Thus, exercise also results in an immediate increase in insulin sensitivity. This increase in insulin sensitivity lasts between 2- 48 hours, depending on the type of exercise.[5]

So far, "exercise" has been mentioned several times, yet it hasn't been defined. Exercise is a physical activity that is structured, planned, and repetitive with the intention of conditioning the body.

The exercises we will be talking about in this chapter consist of cardiovascular training (commonly called "cardio"), strength and resistance training, and flexibility.[6]

Exercise is different from physical activity as physical activity refers to all movements that increase energy use; Physical activity, unlike exercise, is not planned or structured.[7]

To understand how exercise helps control and potentially aids in achieving remission of prediabetes and type 2 diabetes, one must understand the basic biochemistry of the two main types of exercises that have been shown to aid in the control of prediabetes and type 2 diabetes- namely, aerobic and anaerobic exercise.

Aerobic exercise involves the repeated and continuous movement of large muscle groups. Walking, cycling, jogging, and swimming are all different activities that primarily rely on aerobic-energy-producing systems.[8]

"Aerobic" refers to the use of oxygen to adequately meet the energy demands during exercise. During aerobic exercise, one's breathing rate increases to facilitate more oxygen into the lungs. Once the blood has been oxygenated in the lungs, it then moves to the heart and from the heart to the tissues and organs.

At the muscular level, oxygen facilitates the breakdown of fat and carbohydrates to "fuel" the muscles with energy. This is known as oxygen consumption.

Therefore, the more efficient the muscles are at consuming oxygen, the more "fuel" the body can burn, and the more efficient this mechanism is, the longer one can exercise for, and the fitter one becomes.[9]

Aerobic training has been shown to improve insulin sensitivity, lung function, immune function, increase the amount of blood expelled from the heart's ventricles per beat and improve the structural and functional integrity of the blood vessels.

At the cellular level, aerobic exercise has been shown to increase mitochondrial density. The mitochondria are known as "the powerhouse" of the cell.

With an increase in mitochondrial density, the body is able to function more efficiently with less demand for energy. In those with type 2 diabetes, regular aerobic exercise has also been shown to improve HbA1C and blood pressure levels and decrease triglycerides (triglycerides are the fats found in the blood).[10]

Now let's talk about anaerobic exercise. Anaerobic exercise, also known as resistance or strength training, involves brief and intense bursts of physical activity.

Weight lifting, elastic resistance bands, and sprinting are examples of anaerobic exercises.[11]

"Anaerobic" refers to the absence of oxygen. Instead, it is "fueled" by energy already stored in the muscles through a process called glycolysis.

Glycogen, which is the storage form of carbohydrates, is rapidly broken down into glucose through glycolysis. The glucose is then used as a source of energy by the muscles. A by-product of glycolysis is lactic acid production which is responsible for the temporary burning sensation in the muscles that one experiences while doing anaerobic training.[12]

Diabetes is a known and established risk factor for low muscular strength. The benefits of resistance training include increased muscle mass, improved strength, better mental health, improved bone mineral density, improved insulin sensitivity, better blood pressure control, better cardiovascular health, and improved glycemic control.[13]

And finally, flexibility training; flexibility training improves the range of motion around the joints. Exercise activities like yoga and tai chi combine flexibility, balance, and resistance training. Flexibility training is especially important in older individuals with diabetes. As aging has also been associated with reduced joint mobility, and in the presence of hyperglycemia, this is accelerated.

Stretch exercises aid in better joint mobility but don't seem to have an effect on glycemic control. The benefits of yoga and tai chi regarding improved diabetes control are less well established, but they may improve glycemic control.[14]

The Look AHEAD (Action for Health in Diabetes) trial demonstrated that participants had significantly greater and sustained improvements in weight loss, blood glucose control, cardiorespiratory fitness, and blood pressure with a modest energy deficit diet and at least 175 minutes of exercise per week.

These participants also required fewer medications to control their blood glucose levels. The trial also demonstrated that by participating in at least 150 minutes of aerobic exercise per week, there was tighter glycemic control in those with type 2 diabetes.

The trial also concluded that resistance exercises increased strength in adults with type 2 diabetes by about 50% and improved one's HbA1C by about 0.57%.

The trial also found that combining aerobic and anaerobic training was superior to either type of training undertaken alone.[15]

The American Diabetes Association recommends the following when it comes to physical activity and type 2 diabetes[16]:

- Exercising daily or not allowing more than two days to pass between exercise sessions is recommended to enhance insulin action.
- For optimal glycemic and health outcomes, adults

with type 2 diabetes should participate in both
aerobic and anaerobic exercises.

- And in order to prevent or delay the onset of type
  2 diabetes in those that are at a high risk of
  developing type 2 diabetes or have already
  established prediabetes, it is recommended that
  these individuals participate in at least 150 minutes
  of exercise per week and incorporate dietary
  changes which should aim to result in weight loss
  of between 5-7%.

The recommendations mentioned above have
demonstrated a 40-70% risk reduction in developing type 2
diabetes in those with impaired glucose tolerance.[17]

Exercise-induced hypoglycemia (low blood glucose) is
more common in type 1 diabetes. However, to a lesser
extent, it also occurs in those with type 2 diabetes using
insulin and insulin secretagogues (such as glimepiride,
glipizide, repaglinide, and nateglinide).

Unfortunately, when it comes to diabetes, opposites of
complications do tend to occur. The converse of exercise-
induced hypoglycemia, which is known as exercise-
induced hyperglycemia, can also occur.

Exercise-induced hyperglycemia (high blood glucose) is
also more common in type 1 diabetes but has also been
reported in those with type 2 diabetes using insulin.[18]

**Therefore, before starting any exercise regimen, one
must consult with a medical professional. Type 2**

diabetes has also been associated with various cardiovascular complications; therefore, it must be noted again that one should always consult a medical professional before undertaking any new exercise regimen.

Once again, it must be stressed that throughout this book, lifestyle changes are being advocated. And by lifestyle changes, we mean life-long lifestyle changes.

Of course, it is human nature to divert from what we know as the "healthy and right" choices from time to time. However, one cannot expect to achieve remission from prediabetes and type 2 diabetes without seriously changing one's lifestyle.

A Canadian study that assessed the effects of inactivity on health can demonstrate the importance of maintaining a consistently healthy lifestyle.

The study involved overweight, older participants who all had prediabetes. They were told to reduce their step count to less than 1000 steps per day-this roughly equates to the number of steps a housebound individual will take in a day.

At the beginning of the study, their blood glucose levels and insulin sensitivity were monitored and recorded and then again after two weeks of limiting their activity to 1000 steps per day, and then once again after a further two weeks of more physical inactivity.

The study found that the period of inactivity seemed to accelerate the onset of type 2 diabetes. In fact, some of the participants were unable to lower their blood glucose levels despite returning to normal activity levels within the two-week recovery period which followed.

It must be noted that the study did not assess how long it would take or how much extra physical activity may be required for those participants to attain their baseline blood glucose levels and insulin sensitivity. However, this study emphasizes the impact that inactivity can have on blood glucose levels and insulin sensitivity.[19]

Therefore, this study can be used as an example to show how important it is for one to maintain a consistent and healthy lifestyle to control prediabetes and type 2 diabetes and achieve and potentially maintain remission.

A review published in March 2020 in Mayo Clinic Proceedings found that there may be a relationship between the volume of exercise and discontinuation of glucose-lowering medications in the treatment of patients with type 2 diabetes.

The review also noted that this relationship might be dose-dependent. In other words, the more exercise one does, the less medication one may require. However, they also stated that these findings are not conclusive and need more research to make a definitive conclusion.[20]

Not only does regular and vigorous exercise help maintain and potentially aid in achieving remission from prediabetes and type 2 diabetes, but it has also been shown to slow, stop and potentially reverse long-term complications that are associated with type 2 diabetes.

We will now take a look at some of the more apparent benefits of exercise:

Exercise improves vascular health. During exercise, muscles release various substances that benefit vascular and circulatory health. Exercise improves blood flow. And with improved blood flow, tissues and organs have a better supply of oxygen and nutrients.

The improved oxygen and nutrient supply to the tissues and organs aids in reducing the risk of diabetes-associated neuropathy, vision loss, and heart disease. It is also thought that improved blood flow may also aid in better joint health.[21]

Exercise also decreases inflammation. Systemic inflammation is believed to play a significant role in the progression of type 2 diabetes. Always remember that as type 2 diabetes progresses, the risk of developing complications associated with type 2 diabetes also increases.

Due to exercise's anti-inflammatory effects, it is believed that regular exercise can reduce the risks associated with chronic inflammation. Complications include atherosclerosis, cognitive decline, and deterioration of joints.[22]

By exercising, one also improves their cholesterol and blood pressure. As discussed earlier in this chapter, exercise has been shown to decrease LDL "bad cholesterol" levels and increase HDL "good cholesterol" levels.

We also discussed the positive effect exercise has on blood vessels. Exercise also facilitates improved blood flow and reduces chronic inflammation, which strengthens the heart.[23]

It also restores nerve function. For example, a study showed that with just ten weeks of exercise, participants significantly reduced their diabetes-associated pain and neuropathy.[24]

Another benefit of exercise is that it improves joint health. Nerve damage, arterial disease, and excess body weight are all believed to have a significant role in diabetes-associated joint pain.

As we have just discussed, exercise combats all of those mentioned above. Therefore, it is thought that exercise may also aid in improving diabetes-associated joint complications.[25]

To recap, during an exercise session, the muscles demand more glucose for energy. The muscles then take up glucose with minimal insulin action. Therefore, during exercise, the demand for insulin from the pancreas is lowered, and the pancreas essentially does not have to work as hard.

Even after an exercise session, the insulin that the pancreas produces behaves more efficiently. Therefore, the pancreas does not have to work as hard to produce more insulin as exercise has facilitated better and improved insulin sensitivity.

The improved insulin sensitivity then lasts for a couple of hours. Remember, the more vigorous the exercise, the longer the improved insulin sensitivity lasts. In essence, exercise improves the ease at which muscles take up glucose. Therefore, exercise aids in weight loss and weight control, provided that one is following a healthy eating plan.

As we have discussed repeatedly, excess weight and obesity are important risk factors for developing prediabetes and type 2 diabetes.[26]

High-intensity aerobic exercises have been linked to reducing the amount of fat in and around the organs. Remember that excess fat in the liver and pancreas is associated with prediabetes and type 2 diabetes.

High-intensity aerobic exercises also burn lots of calories and therefore facilitate weight loss. And anaerobic exercises, also known as resistance and strength training, basically "suck" up the glucose from the blood when muscles are contracted.[27]

For the reasons mentioned above, the American Diabetes Association recommends participating in both aerobic and anaerobic exercises.

The American Diabetes Association recommends that adults with type 2 diabetes participate in at least 150 minutes of moderate-to-intensely vigorous physical activity a week-of course, combining aerobic and anaerobic exercises.

The 150 minutes of exercise should ideally be spread out over three days, and no more than two consecutive days should pass by in between exercise sessions.

They have also stated that 75 minutes per week of exercise is sufficient if one participates in high-intensity exercises. And they also say that resistance and strength training should ideally be performed on non-consecutive days.[28]

Even though one may have a tremendous structured exercise program, which fulfills all the recommendations by the American Diabetes Association, spending too much time sitting has also been shown to increase weight gain and waist circumference, raise triglyceride levels, and increase blood pressure. All of which are associated with prediabetes and Type 2 diabetes.

Therefore, it is recommended that one should not sit for longer than 30 minutes at a time. One should "take a break" every 30 minutes-even if it just involves stretching or walking to get some water. Even while watching television, avoid lying on the couch for a continuous period and try to "get moving" now and again.[29]

All of this information may seem overwhelming, and one may not even know where to begin. Well, the first step to starting any exercise regime is to understand why exercise is so important.

This chapter has discussed, continuously recapped, and brought forward enough evidence to demonstrate the importance of exercise in those with prediabetes and type 2 diabetes.

Now that we understand the power of regular exercise. Here are some other tips for you to get started with a structured exercise regimen. Please note that one must ensure that one's exercise regimen incorporates the elements recommended by the American Diabetes Association[30]:

- Firstly, **before beginning any exercise endeavor, consult with a trusted medical professional**. This will help ensure that the exercise regimen that one has chosen is well suited for coexisting health conditions that one may have, such as heart disease or diabetic neuropathy.
- Blood glucose monitoring is essential, especially when first starting a new exercise regimen. In this chapter, we discussed that exercise could result in hypoglycemia or hyperglycemia. Therefore, one needs to feel what effect exercise may have on one's blood glucose so that one can adjust their eating habits or insulin dosages accordingly-**under the supervision of a medical professional!**
- Don't go all out. If one is new to exercise, start slowly and with less intensity. Consider starting with exercising for 45 minutes per week and gradually work your way up to 150 minutes per

week. It is okay to start slowly; after all, one must begin somewhere.

- Not all exercise and physical activity have to take place in the form of a structured workout. For example, consider walking instead of driving-especially while running errands. Cleaning the house also counts as physical activity.
- Start with low-impact exercises, especially if one has diabetic neuropathy. Low-impact exercises include stationary cycling, swimming, and weight-bearing exercises. In these instances, one should ease themselves into higher-impact exercises.
- Large muscle group exercises result in maximum benefits.
- Regarding resistance training, multi-joint exercises like squats, lunges, and rows have the most significant benefit.

Research has shown that it takes an average of 66 days to form a new habit-it may take shorter than 66 days for some and longer than 66 days for others.[31]

So, after all, that's been said, how does one ensure that one sticks to an exercise regimen? Well, the best way to do this is to make exercise a habit.

Do something you enjoy: ensure that aerobic and anaerobic exercises are incorporated into your workout programs. For example, if you don't enjoy jogging, try stationary cycling. If you don't enjoy free-weight lifting, try using elastic resistance bands. Exercise is not a punishment. Sure, it may be uncomfortable-especially at first-but you'll soon come to enjoy exercising.[32]

Set aside time for exercising: plan ahead and exercise at the most convenient time for you. Try and stick to these times to make exercising a habit.[33]

Trial and error: use the process of trial and error to find out which exercises you enjoy the most. Perhaps you enjoy exercising alone or find it more motivating to exercise in a group setting.[34]

Plan your exercise program: plan what type of exercises you will do on a particular day. This way, you will be more motivated and more goal-orientated.[35]

Workout clothes: workout clothes are a "uniform," and once you have them on, you'll have an "exercise" mindset.[36]

Discipline: even if you don't feel like working out, workout anyway. However, if you are feeling sick, perhaps skip it until you are feeling better.[37]

Exercising for a reason: your reason for exercising is to help you control your blood glucose level and become healthier. Always keep this in mind.[38]

Accountability: take accountability. Consider having an "accountability partner."[39]

Throughout this chapter, we have discussed the power of regular exercise and how to make exercise a habit. We all know that forming a new habit takes time. For some, exercise may even seem like a form of punishment.

However, if one is disciplined and motivated, it will be just a matter of time before the exercise becomes a part of one's daily life. Always remember the Cooper philosophy; "It is easier to maintain good health through proper exercise, diet, and emotional balance than to regain it once it is lost."

In the next chapter, we will discuss the importance of hydration and water. First, we will explore the importance of water and how water serves the body, especially in diabetes.

Next, we will look at the impact of dehydration and the effects that caffeine, sodas, diet sodas, and alcohol have on the body. Ultimately, we will discover why water is the most superior fluid of all.

THE SECRETS OF HYDRATION-AND HOW TO DO IT RIGHT

I n chapter 6, we discussed the importance of regular exercise. We explored aerobic and anaerobic exercises and concluded that one is not superior to the other.

We discovered that aerobic and anaerobic exercise have a symbiotic relationship when it comes to controlling and even potentially achieving remission from prediabetes and type 2 diabetes.

We brought forward evidence of why it is important to make exercise a habit. We looked at the Canadian trial, whereby older individual's step counts were reduced to 1000 steps per day over two weeks.

The study proved that consistent and regular exercise is required to help control type 2 diabetes. We also discussed the recommendations for exercise made by the

American Diabetes Association, which recommended that individuals with prediabetes and type 2 diabetes should participate in at least 150 minutes of combined aerobic (cardio) and anaerobic (resistance or strength training) exercises per week.

This chapter will now look at the secrets of hydration and how to do it right. It is fair to state that we all know that drinking water is essential. It is also fair to say that water is a crucial nutrient, and its absence in one's diet will prove lethal within a few days.[1]

Many individuals have been lost or abandoned and have managed to survive for days to weeks without food, simply because they have had access to clean, running water.

Even though most of us know that water and hydration are essential, we simply do not know precisely why it is necessary.

In this chapter, we will explore the concept of hydration and why water is necessary. We will also explore why water and hydration are essential in controlling and potentially achieving remission from prediabetes and type 2 diabetes.

In healthy adults, total body water represents an average of 59% for men and 56% for females according to their body mass. However, there are large variations in total body water across and within age groups.[2]

For example, in infants, water comprises about 75% of their body weight, whereas, in the elderly, water comprises about 55% of their body weight.[3] Hence, infants and the elderly are more sensitive to changes in total body water.

Now let's talk about the journey of water once it enters the body; water is distributed within two compartments of the human body; the intracellular compartment and the extracellular compartment.

The intracellular compartment, which refers to the space within the body's cells, contains about 55% of the body's total water. The extracellular compartment is then further subdivided into the intravascular fluid compartment (which is the fluid component of blood) and the interstitial fluid compartment (which is the fluid found around the cells).[4]

The extracellular fluid compartment comprises about 1/3 of the total body water. These relatively high amounts of fluids are constantly being recycled, and equilibrium is only attained and maintained when fluid intake matches fluid loss.[5]

Water intake is derived from two primary sources; directly through drinking fluids and indirectly through eating food substances with high water content, such as certain fruits and vegetables.

As water makes its way through the gastrointestinal system, it is absorbed, and at that level, it also aids in the digestion of other nutrients and as a defense from pathogens. However, there is also "fluid loss" in the gastrointestinal system in the form of secretions from pancreatic juices, bile, gastric secretion, and saliva.

Therefore, at this level, where there is constant fluid loss and fluid absorption, a state of equilibrium must be maintained between intestinal water secretion and intestinal water absorption. If there is a disruption to this state of balance, this is when diarrhea or constipation occurs.[6]

Water is absorbed mainly in the small intestine and to a lesser extent than absorbed in the large intestine. To put this into perspective, if one ingests a total of 8L of water, about 6.5L will be absorbed in the small intestine, while only about 1.3L will be absorbed in the large intestine.[7]

Water and the body's fluids serve several vital functions crucial for the body's optimal functioning. These functions include aiding in the digestion, absorption, and transport of other nutrients, helping maintain the structural and functional integrity of cells, aiding in the removal of waste products and toxins, acting as a medium for biochemical reactions, aiding in thermoregulation, and helping in maintaining lubrication of cavities and joints.

New evidence suggests that bodily fluids may also significantly influence hormone release, cell proliferation, and even cell death.[8]

The human body is constantly in a state of new repair. For the body to "repair" itself, it must first rid itself of old, damaged, and poorly functioning cells, hence cell death. And for the body to replace these old cells, the body must produce newer cells, hence cell proliferation.

Now that one understands the function and importance of water and hydration, one needs to understand the effects of the converse of hydration, which is dehydration, to fully comprehend water's necessity and importance.

- Dehydration of as little as 2% has been shown to have adverse effects on athlete's performances. It has been shown that even under the effects of "mild" dehydration, athletes tended to have decreased endurance, increased fatigue, altered thermoregulatory capability, reduced motivation, and increased perceived effort. However, all of this was mitigated by rehydration.[9] Therefore, this proves that water and hydration are essential for optimal physical performance.
- Dehydration may also influence cognitive performance. Studies have suggested that even mild dehydration may impair concentration, alertness, and short-term memory in children, young adults, and the elderly. Mild to moderate dehydration may also impair arithmetic ability, psychomotor skills, and visuomotor tracking. However, more research is needed on the effects of dehydration on cognitive performance to make a unanimous conclusion.
- Dehydration is also associated with delirium,

which refers to a change in a mental state exhibited by worsening or new-onset confusion, change in the level of consciousness, and even hallucinations. The elderly are particularly at risk of developing delirium. There are many causes and contributing factors that may result in delirium, but out of those many causes, dehydration is one of the leading ones.

- Continuous and persistent dehydration also affects the kidneys. The kidneys play a vital role in regulating and maintaining water equilibrium. Prolonged dehydration causes the kidneys to work harder to maintain a state of water equilibrium. Eventually, the kidneys may not be able to cope with the workload. This may ultimately result in what is known as acute kidney injury. Prolonged dehydration has also been linked to kidney stone formation.[10]

- Dehydration also affects the function of the heart and blood. When fluid levels decrease, so does the circulating blood volume, which leads to hypotension. In severe cases, this can also lead to an emergency condition known as a hypovolemic shock.[11]

- Furthermore, dehydration affects the normal functioning of the gastrointestinal system as water is needed for gut motility and health, and dehydration may also result in constipation. And can damage the gut cells, which can lead to alterations in digestion.[12]

- Dehydration can also cause dryness and "cracking" of the skin. Remember, the skin is the largest organ of the body. And "cracking" of the skin can act as a portal for pathogens.
- Dehydration also causes headaches, migraines, and prolonged migraines. It is postulated that this, in part, is due to intracranial dehydration. It has been shown that in these cases, rehydration with water abates these attacks.[13]

WHAT ARE THE SYMPTOMS OF DEHYDRATION?

The symptoms of dehydration include headache, thirst, dry eyes and mouth, dizziness, tiredness, and concentrated yellow urine. Symptoms of severe dehydration are more problematic and include sunken eyes, low blood pressure, increased heart rate, confusion, and lethargy.[14]

On the other hand, good hydration has been associated with reducing constipation, exercise-induced asthma, hyperglycemia in diabetic ketoacidosis, urinary tract infections, hypertension, coronary heart disease, DVT, and cerebral infarcts (stroke). However, more research needs to be conducted to confirm the above.[15]

So far, we have discussed water, hydration, and dehydration without much reference to prediabetes and type 2 diabetes. Next, we will discuss the importance of hydration with reference to diabetes.

A hormone known as vasopressin or antidiuretic hormone (ADH) is partly responsible for conserving water in the body when the body is not receiving enough water. To put it simply, antidiuretic is released when there is a disruption in water equilibrium. The ultimate aim of antidiuretic is in its name itself-"antidiuretic." Diuresis refers to urination. Therefore, "antidiuresis" means "against" urination.

A paper published by the American Diabetes Association found that increased water intake was associated with lower blood glucose levels.

The article concluded that this was partly due to the effects of vasopressin. Vasopressin receptors are found in several organs, including the kidneys, liver, and the pancreas.

When vasopressin acts on the liver, it is known to induce glucose production and release it into the blood, hence raising blood glucose levels. In a state of good hydration, there is almost no need for vasopressin.

However, in a state of poor hydration, vasopressin is needed to help conserve water. Therefore, vasopressin is released and acts on the kidneys, liver, pancreas, and other organs.

Vasopressin results in antidiuresis and results in the release of glucose from the liver. This is one way dehydration increases blood glucose levels and is detrimental for people with diabetes.[16]

Another way is that dehydration causes glucose in the blood to become more concentrated. This is because water contributes significantly to the intravascular compartment, and the intravascular compartment is made up of blood and fluid.

This increased concentration of glucose in the blood, relative to water deficit, leads to hyperglycemia. In fact, even mild dehydration can raise blood glucose levels by 1.3-2.6 mmol/L (50-100mg/dL).[17]

To make matters even more tedious and confusing, hyperglycemia induces polyuria which means excessive urine output, and this happens due to "glucose-induced osmotic diuresis."

This means that excess glucose in the blood impairs the reabsorption of water and fluids in the blood. And this manifests as increased urination.

The aim of this mechanism, whereby there is increased urination, is to ultimately rid the blood of excess glucose through urine. This diuresis abates when blood glucose levels begin to normalize.

In this situation, blood glucose levels can normalize in two ways: the action of the kidneys ridding the blood of excess glucose through urine or by drugs like insulin. In these instances, one can help the kidneys alleviate the blood of excess glucose by drinking water.

Polyuria is one of the cardinal signs of diabetes. Only once there is adequate control of blood glucose will polyuria abate.[18]

This is also why having uncontrolled diabetes increases the risk of even mild dehydration in people with diabetes.

As we have continuously discussed throughout this book, hyperglycemia leads to increased insulin release from the pancreas.[19] And that increased production and release of insulin from the pancreas for an extended period of time has many consequences, including B-cell exhaustion and increased insulin resistance.

It is thought that increased water intake leads to weight loss in those with prediabetes and type 2 diabetes, which is excellent news.

As we have discussed repeatedly throughout this book, excess fat in the pancreas and liver is partly responsible for prediabetes and type 2 diabetes. This is why the American Diabetes Association recommends weight loss of 5-7% of one's total body weight in individuals with prediabetes and type 2 diabetes.

Theories behind why increased water intake leads to weight loss are as follows[20]:

- Drinking more water means that one is less likely to drink other sugary beverages. Sugary beverages are loaded with unwanted and unnecessary carbohydrates.
- Improved hydration has also been linked to boosting the metabolism. A faster-functioning metabolism means that more calories are burnt- remember that calories are a form of stored

potential energy that the body can use when there is an increased demand for energy.

- Drinking more water may also result in fewer cravings. Most of the time, we crave "unhealthy" foods, and of course, the only way to suppress these cravings is to eat what we are craving. Simply put, if one doesn't crave, one is less likely to indulge in unhealthy foods.
- Diet sodas have been linked to increased insulin resistance. However, if one replaces diet soda with water, at least partially, to begin with, the likelihood of insulin resistance is decreased.

Throughout this chapter, we have discussed the importance of maintaining a good state of hydration through drinking water. However, in some individuals, increasing their water intake may be detrimental to their health.

Those with kidney disease and related conditions, thyroid disease, liver disease, heart conditions, those that use medications that encourage water retention, those that chronically use NSAIDs (non-steroidal anti-inflammatory drugs), those that use certain antidepressants, and those that use opiate-based medications should consult a medical professional before suddenly increasing their water intake.[21]

As stated repeatedly, throughout this book, before committing to starting any "new" lifestyle, one should always seek the opinion of a medical professional.

Throughout this chapter, we have discussed water and hydration as a single entity. It must be stressed that not just any fluid one drinks will aid in good hydration. Many other liquids do not facilitate maintaining a good state of hydration; in fact, they may even worsen prediabetes and type 2 diabetes.

Let us take a look at what one should avoid, especially for people with diabetes.

Caffeine: It has been shown that consuming large amounts of caffeine, which is found abundantly in coffee and energy drinks, worsens insulin resistance. Caffeine also increases acid production in the stomach, leading to heartburn and even an "upset" stomach.

Due to its effects on the digestive system, caffeine also impairs calcium absorption and metabolism, leading to osteoporosis. Caffeine also increases urination and blood pressure. We are not saying that one should completely cut coffee out, but we strongly urge one to be cautious when it comes to excess caffeine intake.[22]

Diet Soda: Although diet sodas may seem to be a healthier alternative to sugar-sweetened sodas, they are not. In fact, both diet sodas and sugar-sweetened sodas are not advised in those with prediabetes and type 2 diabetes. This is because diet sodas are loaded with artificial sweeteners. Studies have shown that artificial sweeteners harm the normal gut flora in the digestive system, increase insulin resistance, and cause weight gain.[23]

Alcohol: Alcohol causes blood glucose levels to decrease, and this can last up to 12 hours. When this effect is combined with glucose-lowering medications, this can be disastrous and can lead to hypoglycemia. Alcohol is metabolized in the liver, and one of the liver's primary functions is to regulate blood glucose.

While the liver is metabolizing alcohol, it may not effectively control blood glucose levels, resulting in hypoglycemia.[24] One may think that drinking alcoholic beverages loaded with carbohydrates will help counteract hypoglycemia; unfortunately, it's just not that simple.

Liquid sugars (glucose) are absorbed quickly in the body, offering no protection from hypoglycemia in the upcoming hours. However, food is digested at a slower rate, which offers some form of protection from hypoglycemia, hence why one should never drink alcohol on an empty stomach.[25]

ALCOHOL CONSUMPTION IS ALSO A LEADING CAUSE OF CANCER; CANCER RESEARCH UK STATES THAT[26]:

- Alcohol is a possible cause of several types of cancers.
- What type of alcohol you drink does not matter; it's the alcohol content that counts.
- Whatever your drinking habits, cut it down and drink water instead; it will help you reduce your risk.

If you consume alcohol, the chance is that you are more likely to get cancer, but that doesn't mean it's set in stone and you are guaranteed to become a cancer patient in the future, your risk will depend on many things, some of which you have no power over, e.g., your genetics and your age.[27]

However, cutting back or giving up has many benefits, from reducing your chance of developing cancers such as breast cancer, bowel cancer, throat cancer, mouth cancer, having an accident, having liver disease to protecting yourself from high blood pressure.[28]

Alcohol consumption can cause cancer in three ways[29]:

Cell damage: after consuming alcohol, the body turn's that alcohol into a chemical known as acetaldehyde. This chemical destroys the cells and halts them from repairing the damage that drinking alcohol has caused.

Change to your hormones: alcohol has the power to change the levels of hormones such as insulin and estrogen; the higher the levels of these hormones in our body, the greater the chance that the hormones will make the cells divide, which in turn raises the opportunity for cancer cells to develop.

Change to the cells of the throat and mouth: the cells in our mouths and throats change due to alcohol consumption, and when this happens, they allow for the absorption of harmful chemicals, if any of those harmful chemicals are cancer-causing chemicals like those found in the smoke of cigarettes, they can cause some severe damage.

After hearing the above, I think it's safe to say that one will only be doing their body's a huge favor by giving up alcohol.

According to the American Diabetes Association, a woman should not drink more than one serving of alcohol per day. At the same time, men should not consume more than two servings of alcohol per day. A serving is defined as 340ml (12 ounces) of beer, 142ml (5 ounces) of wine, or 43ml (1.5 ounces) of distilled spirits.[30]

It must also be stressed that regularly consuming high-carbohydrate-containing alcohol may lead to weight gain.

When it comes to alcohol, there are a few "tips" to be aware of in those with prediabetes and type 2 diabetes[31]:

- One should avoid low-sugar beers and ciders. These types of drinks are also called "diabetic drinks." They may contain fewer carbohydrates, but they do generally have more alcohol.
- One should also avoid low-alcohol wines. Even though they may contain less alcohol, they generally have more carbohydrates.
- Try and opt for water as a mixer rather than sugar-containing mixers. Some "sugar-free" mixers may contain artificial sweeteners.
- Spirits, dry wines, and prosecco contain fewer carbohydrates than beers, ales, and ciders.

Although water is the best way to stay hydrated, there are some other alternatives-after all, only drinking water can become rather tiresome. Unsweetened tea and flavored water are better alternatives to coffee, sodas, and diet sodas.[32] However, one should always be mindful of why water is the most superior fluid of them all.

The American Diabetes Association states that a diabetic's daily water intake requirement is the same as a healthy person's unless otherwise specified by a personal physician. The Institute of Medicine also suggests that women should drink about 2.2 liters of fluid per day, and men should drink about 3 liters of fluid per day.

"Fluid" refers to water and herbal teas and not carbonated, caffeinated, or artificially-sweetened drinks.[33]

One of the easiest ways to track how much water one drinks is to fill a one-liter bottle with water and refill it throughout the day. Instead of reaching for a soda, go for the bottle of water.

We have discussed and explored the concept of hydration and why water is a vital yet undervalued nutrient. We have seen why water is the best option to "quench" one's thirst and have proven why people have been able to stay alive for days to weeks by just having access to clean, running water.

As mentioned repeatedly throughout this chapter, there simply is no better replacement for water when it comes to hydration.

In the next chapter, we will explore the importance of sleep. We will discuss the two main sleep phases, rapid eye movement (REM) and non-rapid eye movement (NREM). We will discover the hormonal effects that sleep deprivation has on the body and discuss the concept of sleep hygiene. We will also look at techniques that one can use for better sleep hygiene.

8

SLEEP: THE FORGOTTEN
COMPONENT OF GOOD HEALTH

In the previous chapter, we discussed the importance of hydration. We discovered that total body water represents an average of 59% for men and 56% for females according to their body mass.

We discussed the importance of water and how water helps aid in the digestion, absorption, and transport of other nutrients and helps maintain the structural and functional integrity of cells, aids in the removal of waste products and toxins, acts as a medium for biochemical reactions, aids in thermoregulation and helps in maintaining lubrication of cavities and joints.

We also discussed dehydration and how even mild dehydration can impact one's day-to-day functioning and activities.

Next, we looked at how water aids in helping and controlling blood glucose levels. Finally, we discussed the effects of caffeine, sodas, diet sodas, and alcohol on the body. Ultimately, we concluded that water is the most superior fluid of all.

This chapter will now look at a forgotten component for good health, which is sleep.

Sleep can be defined as "an active state of unconsciousness produced by the body where the brain is in a relative state of rest and is reactive primarily to internal stimulus."

Sleep is an extremely complicated process, and its exact purpose has not yet been demystified. There are several theories exploring the functions and importance of sleep. However, the most prominent ones are the inactive theory, energy conservation theory, restoration theory, and brain plasticity theory.[1]

- **Inactive theory:** this theory is based on the concept of evolutionary pressure whereby it was safer to be inactive at night, in the dark, from predators.
- **Energy conservative theory:** this theory is based on the fact that one's metabolism decreases by up to 10% during sleep. Therefore, the primary function of sleep is to reduce one's energy demand during that part of day and night when it is less efficient to hunt.
- **Restorative theory:** this theory is based on the fact that muscle repair, tissue growth, protein

synthesis, and release of many vital hormones for growth occur primarily during sleep. Therefore, according to the restorative theory, sleep enables the body to repair itself and replenish cellular components which are necessary for normal functioning. However, these cellular components need replacing after they become depleted during the awake cycle.

- **Brian plasticity theory:** this theory states that sleep is essential for neural recognition and growth of the brain's structure and function. This theory looks to the development of the brain in infants and children and explains why infants must sleep for at least 14 hours per day.

The basis of all of these theories is reasonable and logical. Therefore, it is acceptable to conclude that the importance and function of sleep are not based on one theory alone but rather a combination of all of these theories. The simple fact of the matter is that sleep is essential-no matter which approach one favors.

As stated previously, sleep is a complicated process. In fact, sleep involves multiple areas of the brain. Some of the areas in the brain involved in sleep include the hypothalamus, the thalamus, and the pons.

The hypothalamus contains an area which is known as the body's "biological clock." Both the thalamus and the hypothalamus regulate deep sleep. In addition, the pons has a vital role in regulating rapid eye movement (REM) sleep. We'll get to the importance and significance of deep sleep and REM sleep later on.[2]

The structures mentioned above need to be regulated-if they weren't, sleep would become somewhat hazardous. The mechanisms that control sleep are of 2 types; sleep / wake homeostasis and the circadian rhythm.

Homeostasis refers to the principles of equilibrium and balance of the body.[3] And the circadian rhythm are 24-hour cycles that are part of the body's "internal clock." They regulate both mental and physical systems. One of the most well-known circadian rhythms is, in fact, the sleep / wake cycle.

The circadian rhythm of the body is connected to a "master clock." This master clock is located in the brain within the hypothalamus-remember we just discussed the importance of the thalamus and the hypothalamus with regards to deep sleep.

This area, within the hypothalamus, is highly sensitive to light. When this area mentioned above is triggered, it activates "clock genes," which send signals to regulate activity throughout the body.

During the day, when there is light, the "master clock" sends signals that generate alertness. As night falls, when there is less light, the "master clock" initiates melatonin production.

Melatonin is a hormone that promotes sleep. During sleep, it keeps on transmitting signals to maintain sleep.[4] As the sleep/wake homeostasis keeps track of the body's need for sleep, it also reminds the body to sleep after a certain amount of time and regulates sleep intensity. The mechanism also causes longer and deeper sleep after a period of sleep deprivation.[5]

Believe it or not, there are also phases of sleep. The two main phases of sleep are:

- Rapid eye movement sleep (REM) and
- Non-rapid eye movement sleep (NREM).

There is a cycle between these two sleep phases. They sequentially rotate between five to six times during the night, which generally lasts between 90 and 100 minutes between rotations.[6]

Rapid eye movement, dreaming, decreased muscle tone, and sleep paralysis all occur during REM sleep.[7]

NREM sleep is a bit more complicated than REM sleep. In fact, it is further divided into three different stages of increasing sleep depth.

Sleep stage 1 refers to the transitional phase between sleep and wakefulness. It refers to the stage when one "drifts off" to sleep, which generally lasts around 5-10 minutes.

Sleep stage 2 refers to the onset of sleep and lasts for approximately 20 minutes. During this stage, the heart rate slows down, and there is a drop in body temperature.

Finally, sleep stage 3 is referred to as deep sleep. This stage lasts between 20-40 minutes. During this stage, the muscles relax, the rate of breathing slows down, blood pressure drops, and one becomes less responsive to external stimuli.[8]

Earlier on, we mentioned that during sleep, essential hormones are released. These hormones include melatonin, follicle-stimulating hormone (FSH), luteinizing hormone (LH), and growth hormone.[9]

- Melatonin is vital in regulating biological rhythms (such as sleep) and the immune system.[10]
- FSH and LH both play critical roles in the reproductive system.[11]
- And the growth hormone is essential in physical growth and maturation.[12]

Now that we have discussed sleep basics, let us discuss the relationship between sleep and type 2 diabetes.

Studies have found a higher risk of developing obesity and type 2 diabetes when individuals sleep less than 5-6 hours per night and have poor sleep quality. Conversely, studies have also reported higher risks of developing obesity and type 2 diabetes in individuals who sleep longer than 9 hours per night.

The categories of sleep disturbance that leads to increased risk include alternations of sleep duration (which include both chronic sleep restriction and excessive sleep), alterations in sleep architecture (sleep architecture refers to the two phases of sleep; REM and NREM sleep), sleep fragmentation (this refers to the interruptions of sleep), circadian rhythm disorders and disturbances (for example this occurs in shift workers) and obstructive sleep apnea (OSA).[13]

In fact, a recent review of data demonstrated that sleep disturbances might be as significant a risk factor as traditional risk factors for the development of diabetes. The study further revealed that difficulty in initiating sleep increased the risk of developing type 2 diabetes by 55%, while difficulty in maintaining sleep increased its risk by 74%.[14]

One may be wondering how sleep disturbances contribute to the development of type 2 diabetes. Well, sleep disturbances are associated with the dysregulation of the neuroendocrine control of appetite.

It is thought that sleep deprivation also leads to hyperactivity of the orexin system. Orexin is a chemical in the brain that regulates arousal, wakefulness, and hunger.

There is also an increase in ghrelin, a hunger-promoting hormone, and a decrease in circulating leptin, a hormone that contributes to one feeling full and satisfied after eating.[15]

Poor sleep also induces cravings for high-fat and high-sugar-containing foods. It also causes the brain's reward center to go into overdrive. Interestingly, insufficient sleep has also been associated with impulsive behavior and decreased ability to make complex judgments and decision making.[16]

All of the above-mentioned causes one to overeat. For example, one study suggested that poor sleep can lead to eating 385 extra calories per day. In addition, those who have an inadequate sleep are more likely to eat at night, which also contributes to disrupting the circadian rhythm.

Poor sleep is also known to make one sedentary due to lack of energy. Therefore, one is less likely to exercise.[17] Remember, the American Diabetes Association recommends that those with prediabetes and type 2 diabetes participate in at least 150 minutes of anaerobic and aerobic exercise per week to control their glucose levels. Refer back to chapter 6 to recap the importance of exercise.

All of the points mentioned above contribute to weight gain. Those with prediabetes and type 2 diabetes should aim for a weight loss of 5-7%, according to the American Diabetes Association, which has been discussed in detail in chapter 6.

Now, it is possible that one is participating in clean and healthy eating, exercising and keeping adequately hydrated, and still not losing weight. This may be due to poor sleep hygiene.

Let's take a look at some of the problems one can face when one deprives oneself of sleep.

A study demonstrated that an insulin-resistant state might be induced by sleep deprivation. In another study, it was reported that a one-week period of sleep restriction (only 4 hours of sleep) in young, healthy participants could induce a state of prediabetes. And, it was demonstrated that chronic sleep deprivation was associated with impaired glucose tolerance.

It is thought that sleep fragmentation activates a part of the sympathetic nervous system, which increases blood glucose levels by decreasing insulin sensitivity.[18] In fact, the activation of the sympathetic nervous system may increase circulating levels of cortisol, which is the steroid hormone that causes increased insulin resistance.

Furthermore, insomnia and obstructive sleep apnea (OSA), and restless leg syndrome are common among those with type 2 diabetes. The above-mentioned are well-known risk factors for poor sleep quality and, in fact, sleep disturbances.[19]

Obstructive sleep apnea affects one's ability to breathe at night. As a result, one is constantly being aroused from sleep due to one's inability to breathe. Often, this happens multiple times during sleep. Therefore, one cannot get a good night's sleep and feels excessive sleepiness the next day.

Obstructive sleep apnea is common among those aged 35-54 years and is especially prevalent in overweight people.[20]

Restless leg syndrome is characterized by unpleasant and uncomfortable feelings in the legs. It causes one to move one's legs to rid oneself of the feeling. This feeling of discomfort and movement leads to disruption and disturbance of sleep.[21]

Hypoglycemia is also a risk factor for sleep disturbance, especially in those taking nighttime insulin. Hypoglycemia leads to sleep distribution, difficulty waking up in the morning, and tiredness during the day.[22]

Furthermore, nocturnal polyuria (excessive urination at night due to hyperglycemia) is also a contributing factor to sleep disturbance in diabetics.[23]

Now for the crux of the matter-insulin and its relationship with sleep. At this stage of the book, it is fair to say that insulin is needed for "the proper behavior of glucose." Many studies have shown that poor sleep negatively affects how the body uses insulin.

Studies have also shown that having enough deep sleep is linked with proper blood glucose regulation by insulin. It is important to remember that even though sleep decreases the rate of one's metabolism, the body still requires glucose to fulfill its functions.[24]

It has also been shown that the body requires different amounts of glucose at different stages and phases of sleep. For example, the body needs less glucose during REM sleep. However, during 4 am and 8 am, there is a surge in blood glucose. Therefore, at this stage, insulin is required to prevent hyperglycemia.

Ideally, insulin should be able to function optimally. However, increased insulin resistance in sleep deprivation leads to alterations in one's insulin and glucose levels.[25]

Interestingly, it has been postulated that lack of sleep may induce stress on the pancreas.[26] Insulin is produced and secreted by the pancreas. Suppose there is stress on the pancreatic cells. In that case, they cannot function optimally, which results in the alteration in the production and secretion of insulin, leading to hyperglycemia. Over time, this may also contribute to insulin resistance.

As discussed earlier, lack of sleep also causes an increase in circulating cortisol. In addition, lack of sleep causes alterations to other hormones as well like thyroid-stimulating hormone (TSH) and testosterone. These alterations in other hormones also contribute to increased insulin resistance.[27]

Noticeable signs of sleep deprivation include daytime fatigue, irritability, frequent yawning, and excessive sleepiness. One may think that caffeine may be the answer to overcome this in an acute setting. However, caffeine is never the answer.

Chapter 7 discussed what caffeine does to the body and why it is especially hazardous for prediabetes and type 2 diabetes. Caffeine is a stimulant. Due to this, it can make sleep deprivation worse by making it harder for one to fall asleep at night.[28]

Sleep deprivation wreaks havoc on the body in general, and chronic sleep deprivation leaves the brain exhausted. Sleep is also essential in forming new pathways in the brain, which helps one remember new information.

Chronic sleep deprivation does not allow for this process to occur optimally. As a result, one may find it challenging to concentrate and learn new things. Chronic sleep deprivation also leads to a delay in the signals that the brain sends to the body. This partly manifests as a decrease in coordination which increases one's risk for accidents.[29]

Sleep deprivation also affects one's mental and emotional status. For example, one may feel impatient and become more prone to mood swings. Other psychological features of chronic sleep deprivation include impulsive behavior, anxiety, depression, paranoia, and suicidal thoughts. In addition, if sleep deprivation continues for long enough, one may also start experiencing hallucinations.[30]

During sleep, antibodies and cytokines are produced. These are important for the immune system's function. Therefore, sleep deprivation will also lead to lower immunity.[31]

As stated earlier, sleep deprivation is associated with weight gain due to alterations in brain chemistry. As discussed throughout this book, those with prediabetes and type 2 diabetes should aim for weight loss and not weight gain. In addition, sleep deprivation also alters the production and release of insulin and decreases insulin sensitivity.[32]

Sleep plays an essential role in the body's ability to heal and repair the heart's blood vessels. In fact, sleep deprivation has been associated with an increased risk of heart attack and stroke.[33]

Earlier, we discussed that some hormones are produced and secreted during sleep. The first is testosterone; now, in order for testosterone to be secreted, one needs at least three hours of uninterrupted sleep.

The second is growth hormone; growth hormone is especially important in children and adolescents for growth and maturation-both testosterone and growth hormone aid in building muscle mass and help repair tissues, and interruption in sleep interferes with the function of these hormones.[34]

To get enough sleep and get good quality sleep, one needs to practice good sleep hygiene, which refers to habits conducive to sleeping regularly. It is recommended that adults sleep between 7-9 hours at night.

Here are some tips to help make sleep easier[35]:

- **Exercise:** Exercise helps boost the effects of natural sleep hormones such as melatonin. However, exercising before bedtime can act as a stimulant.

Therefore, try and exercise in the morning or early afternoon.

- **Reserve your bed for sleeping:** To be a stimulus for sleep and not wakefulness, don't use your bed as an office and try to avoid watching late-night television in bed.
- **Tranquility and calmness:** try and make your bedroom comfortable for sleep and relaxation. Ideally, your bedroom should be dark and quiet.
- **Start a sleep ritual:** this will help signal that it's becoming time to sleep to your body and mind. For example, have a relaxing bath or listen to peaceful music. You can do anything that is not overstimulating as a ritual.
- **Eat:** but not too much. Being hungry and being overly full can lead to poor sleep. Try eating dinner at least 2- 3 hours before bedtime.
- **Avoid alcohol and caffeine:** Alcohol and caffeine are both stimulants. Avoid stimulants before bedtime. Also, try and avoid anything which can give you heartburn, like citrus fruits.
- **De-stress:** stress is a stimulant. Before bedtime, allow yourself some time to wind down. Try breathing exercises.
- **Get checked:** if you have an urge to move your legs, snore, or have burning pain in your stomach or chest, you should seek medical advice. This could be due to restless leg syndrome, sleep apnea, or gastroesophageal reflux.

After reading through this chapter, it is fair to say that sleep is a complicated process and has many vital functions. Before reading this chapter, one may have thought that sleep was "just to have more energy for the next day." In part, this is true. But we have discovered that sleep has many more functions than we ever thought.

We have also learned how sleep deprivation leads to not only increased insulin resistance but also hyperglycemia.

After all of the above, we can conclude that one needs to practice good sleep hygiene to experience the positive effects of sleep and ward off the adverse effects of sleep deprivation.

In the next chapter, we will discuss mental health and particularly stress. We will discuss acute stress, episodic acute stress, and chronic stress. We will explore the physiological mechanisms of stress and how it leads to hyperglycemia and reduced immunity. We will also look at strategies on how to recognize and cope with stress.

9

ADDRESSING MENTAL HEALTH: WHY REDUCING STRESS IS CRUCIAL

I n the previous chapter, we discussed sleep and its importance. We discussed the different theories which looked at why sleep is crucial; inactive theory, energy conservation theory, restoration theory, and brain plasticity theory.

We concluded that the importance and function of sleep are not based on one theory alone but rather a combination of all of these theories. We explored some of the areas of the brain which helped regulate sleep and discussed the body's "biological clock."

We also looked at the two systems which regulate sleep; The circadian rhythm and sleep/wake homeostasis. We touched on the two phases of sleep, REM and NREM sleep, and discovered that these two phases cycle between each other every 90-100 minutes.

We explored the link between sleep deprivation and hyperglycemia. We also learned that essential hormones such as growth hormone, melatonin, follicle-stimulating hormone, and luteinizing hormones are secreted during sleep.

Conversely, we discovered how poor sleep leads to interference with hormones such as cortisol and testosterone, contributing to insulin resistance.

Finally, we discussed what sleep hygiene is and the principles of sleep hygiene. Ultimately, we concluded that one needs between 7-9 hours of uninterrupted sleep at night to have proper metabolic and cognitive functioning.

Before we divulge any further into mental health and why reducing Stress Is Crucial, we should look at the definitions and concepts pertaining to mental health.

The WHO (World Health Organization) defines mental health as a "state of balance, both within and with the environment.

Physical, psychological, social, cultural, spiritual and other interrelated factors participate in producing this balance."

The WHO recognizes that "mental health is the foundation for an individual's well-being and effective functioning."

The WHO also states that mental health and physical health are entwined together. Good mental health does not merely mean the absence of a mental disorder. Good mental health enables one to think, learn and understand one's emotions and the reactions of others.[1]

The American Psychological Association defines stress as "any uncomfortable emotional experience accompanied by predictable biochemical, physiological and behavioral changes."[2]

In addition, the American Psychological Association recognizes three forms of stress; acute stress, episodic acute stress, and chronic stress.[3]

Acute stress: This is the most common form of stress. It stems from two sources. One source is from pressures and demands of the recent past. The other source is from anticipated pressures and demands of the near future.

Due to the fact that acute stress is short-term, it is not associated with the extensive and long-term damage that chronic stress is associated with. It is important to note here that not all stress is bad; acute stress can act as a form of motivation to simply get things done. However, "overdoing" short-term stress is not good either. Generally speaking, acute stress is manageable.[4]

Episodic acute stress This is acute stress which occurs in more frequent bouts.[5]

Chronic stress: This is a prolonged and constant feeling of stress. The body remains in a constant state of psychological arousal due to the fact that the "stressors" occur with such frequency and intensity that the autonomic nervous system of the body does not have time to relax.[6]

To understand the complications and side effects of stress, especially emotional stress, one must understand how the body reacts to stress on a biological level. So first, we will discuss the acute stress response and then the chronic stress response.

When the body experiences acute stress, a cascade of events occurs in the nervous, cardiovascular, endocrine (hormones), and immune systems.

Firstly, stress hormones are released to make immediate energy available to the body. Secondly, a new pattern of energy distribution emerges. Energy is diverted to the tissues that are crucial to overcoming the immediate stressor. In other words, tissues that aid in the "fight-or-flight" response. This is an evolutionary protective mechanism.[7]

The brain, skeletal muscles, and the immune system then become "loaded" with energy. However, while these systems become energized, other systems that do not serve a crucial function in the acute stress response, such as the digestive and reproductive systems, have energy diverted away from them.

This response, whereby massive amounts of energy are needed, involves releasing glucose into the blood. Two major stress hormones facilitate this process, epinephrine and cortisol.

In addition, these two stress hormones encourage lipolysis and the conversion of glycogen into glucose. Lipolysis is a metabolic process whereby fats are broken down into usable energy sources like fatty acids and glycerol.[8]

Now that the body has made an immediate form of energy available, the energy needs to quickly get to the tissues and organs, which are crucial in the acute stress's response. Therefore, as a result, one's blood pressure is raised.

Two mechanisms, the myocardial response and the vascular response are responsible for this rise in blood pressure. Specific stressors elicit either one of the mechanisms to occur. Stressors that require one to "do something," such as to give a speech, are associated with what is known as the myocardial response. In essence, the myocardial response results in more blood being expelled out of the heart; hence there is an increase in one's heart rate.

On the other hand, stressors that require more vigilant coping strategies in the absence of movement, such as viewing a distressing video, elicit what is known as the vascular response. The vascular response raises the blood pressure by constricting the blood vessels.

These are both evolutionary responses. From this perspective, the myocardial response actively shunts blood to the skeletal muscles, whereas the vascular response shunts blood away from the periphery to the internal organs.[9]

Finally, with regards to the acute stress response, the immune system becomes activated. Immune cells are released from the lymphatic tissue and spleen into the blood. They then make their way into tissues that are most likely to suffer physical damage during the acute stress response. In this way, the immune cells are now in an optimal position to protect the body from microbes and aid in healing.[10]

Although this chapter is mainly about chronic stress, one needs to fully understand the acute stress response to fully comprehend the effects of chronic stress.

The chronic stress response occurs when the acute stress response has become maladaptive due to repeated or continuous activation. Therefore, the chronic stress response follows the same pathway as the acute stress response, except that its constant activation leads to complications.

Now understand that persistently elevated levels of stress hormones ultimately lead to a sustained increase in blood pressure. And chronically elevated blood pressure (hypertension) is known to cause left ventricular hypertrophy.

Chronically elevated and rapidly shifting blood pressure levels can also damage the arteries and plaque formation. Chronically elevated levels of stress hormones are also known to suppress the immune system and response.

Stress hormones also affect the molecules which communicate with the cells of the immune system. If the immune system cells receive no communication, they simply cannot be mobilized to the affected tissues to protect the body.[11]

Unfortunately, chronic stress affects just about every body system, hence why we dedicated a whole chapter to stress.

Stress has also been shown to affect brain function. The effects of stress on the nervous system, including the brain, have been studied for over 50 years. It has been demonstrated that chronic stress can lead to atrophy (which means wasting away) of the brain and decrease its weight. This ultimately leads to structural changes, which leads to different and altered responses to stress, cognition, and memory.

It must be noted here that the degree and intensity of changes to the brain depend on the level of stress and the duration of stress. There are many structures in the brain that we discovered in the previous chapter.

Each structure has a purpose and function. Most of the structures in the brain have multiple functions. Studies have shown that stress has a significant impact on at least three structures in the brain. These are the hippocampus, amygdala, and temporal lobe.

The hippocampus and amygdala have a crucial function in memory. In addition, the hippocampus, amygdala, and temporal lobe all play a significant role in cognition and learning. Therefore, functional changes that occur in the brain due to stress have been shown to affect long-term memory, spatial memory, verbal memory, cognition, and reaction time. In fact, chronic stress has even been associated with mood disorders.[12]

Stress also affects nutrition and the gastrointestinal system. The effects of stress at this level can be summarized into two aspects.

- The first aspect is that stress affects appetite. This occurs at the level of the brain. Interestingly, stress can either cause an increase in appetite, hence the phrase "stress-eater," or a decrease in appetite.
- The second aspect is that stress adversely affects the normal function of the gastrointestinal system. Studies have shown that stress disrupts the absorption process, mucus and acid secretion, and intestinal permeability.

Stress also sensitizes the gastrointestinal system to inflammation which ultimately may lead to gastrointestinal inflammatory diseases. Stress has also been shown to reactivate dormant inflammatory conditions of the gastrointestinal system. Therefore, Crohn's disease and other ulcerative-based diseases of the gastrointestinal system are associated with stress.

Irritable bowel syndrome (IBS) also has a high association with stress. Stress also affects the gastrointestinal tract movement, resulting in delayed stomach emptying.[13]

Furthermore, stress also affects the endocrine system. The endocrine system controls the production and secretion of hormones. We discussed the role that the endocrine system played when we discussed the acute stress response.

To recap, we discussed how epinephrine and cortisol are released from the adrenal glands during the acute stress response. We also discussed that the production and secretion of hormones are controlled at the level of the brain and results in an axis-type of relationship between the brain and the tissues which secrete the hormones.

It has also been shown that stress can either activate or change the activity of many endocrine processes associated with the adrenal glands, gonads, thyroid, and pancreas.[14]

The effects that stress has on the endocrine system is where the relationship between stress and diabetes lies.

A Swedish study of men born between 1921-1925 found that chronic stress for a period of 1-5 years was associated with a 45% increase in the risk of being diagnosed with either type 1 or type 2 diabetes.[15]

Stress is said to affect the occurrence of prediabetes and type 2 diabetes in two ways.

The first is that one's reaction to stress may induce an unhealthy lifestyle that can manifest as neglecting one's physical well-being in eating unhealthy and not being motivated to exercise. In fact, stress may lead one to eat in a consoling manner-we just discussed the relationship between stress and appetite.

The second is the effect that stress has on the endocrine and immune systems. Earlier on, we discovered that cortisol is released from the adrenal glands to respond to stress.

Psychological strain induces the production and secretion of a cascade of hormones, including cortisol, growth hormones, and epinephrine.

From previous chapters, we know that cortisol encourages the release of glucose from the liver and inhibits insulin action. Therefore, cortisol increases blood glucose levels.

Growth hormone also encourages the release of glucose from the liver and blunts the action of insulin. Therefore, growth hormone also increases blood glucose levels.[16]

Epinephrine, also known as adrenaline, is also released from the adrenal glands. And also promotes the release of glucose from the liver into the blood. Therefore, epinephrine also increases blood glucose levels. Earlier on, we discussed the evolutionary need for increased "more energy" in response to stress. You should know that this energy is in the form of glucose.

When stress becomes constant and chronic, it contributes to a continuous state of hyperglycemia. Therefore, chronic stress can aggravate a prediabetic or type 2 diabetic state.

Throughout this chapter, we have mentioned stress. Although we have defined stress, we haven't discussed what "counts" as stress, also known as "perceived stress."

It is important to note that different individuals perceive stress differently. Stress can be due to work pressure, interpersonal relationships such as marriage, health problems like diabetes itself, financial insecurity, and even traffic.[17]

Because individuals perceive stress differently, individuals react differently to stress. This is especially important to remember in those with anxiety and even type-A personalities. It is especially important to remember here that it is with reference to long-term and chronic stress when we talk about the adverse effects of stress.

The acute stress response is an evolutionary protective mechanism that brings about the "fight-or-flight" response.

It must be noted that even "happy stressors" such as planning a wedding or getting a job promotion result in the "fight-or-flight" response. This also affects one's blood glucose levels.

In those with diabetes, it is vital to keep track of one's blood glucose levels in any stress, whether it is "happy" stress or not.

As discussed previously, stress is known to induce an unhealthy lifestyle. This manifests in eating a poor-quality diet, decreased exercise, smoking, and excessive alcohol consumption.[18]

We have discussed the effects of an unhealthy diet, alcohol consumption, and exercise on prediabetes and type 2 diabetes. It is important to remember that at some stage in one's life, one will experience stress. However, it is also important to remember that, especially during stress, one should lead a healthy and active lifestyle to try and overcome the hormonal effects of chronic stress.

Stress manifests itself in many different forms. In acute stress situations, one may experience anxiousness, nervousness, distraction, worry, and pressure.

When stress levels increase or occur for a more extended period of time, one may experience fatigue, depression, chest pain or anxiety, rapid heartbeat, dizziness, difficulty breathing, menstrual cycle irregularities, erectile dysfunction, and loss of libido. Stress may also lead to poor sleep hygiene and loss of appetite or overeating.[19]

Ironically, stress itself interferes with one's ability to self-manage diabetes. For example, research has shown that doing everyday self-care tasks such as monitoring glucose frequently, following a meal plan, and correctly taking insulin or oral hypoglycemic drugs becomes difficult during times of stress.[20]

The American Diabetes Association recognizes this phenomenon as "diabetes burnout." The American Diabetes Association states that "with diabetes, feeling physically good is half the battle. Feeling mentally good is the other half."[21]

One needs to recognize when one is stressed, but more important is one's approach to dealing with stress; there are multiple ways one can deal with stress[22]:

- **By monitoring one's blood glucose.** We discussed the physiological mechanism of stress and how it raises one's blood glucose levels. Therefore, it is extremely important during stress that one tracks their blood glucose levels more vigilantly. Then, **with the help of a medical professional**, one can make adjustments. Also, during these times, it is more crucial than ever that one follows an active and healthy lifestyle.
- **By informing your doctor.** It is important to inform one's healthcare team of "good" and "bad" stress. Earlier, we discussed that the body doesn't distinguish between "good" and "bad" stress. Instead, the body perceives stress as stress and acts accordingly. One's healthcare team will adjust treatments and offer advice on coping through a stressful period.
- **By re-evaluating.** One should re-evaluate the causes of their long-term stressors. Are these stressors worth it, and more importantly, is one able to adjust them? For example, if work is the cause of long-term stress, perhaps one should consider changing one's working environment.
- **By getting rid of accumulated short-term stressors.** Although short-term stressors are not as detrimental as long-term stressors, the accumulation of minor infringements on one's life can amount. Therefore, one should try and limit one's interaction with minor stressors. For example, if traffic is a constant annoyance, try and

leave for work a little earlier to avoid traffic or use public transport.

- **By cooling-off.** One must develop mechanisms to help destress. This could involve reading books, going for a massage, sitting in the garden, listening to music, talking to a friend, or seeking professional help.
- **By practicing mindfulness.** A study found that those who practiced mindfulness-based stress reduction techniques showed improved fasting blood glucose and HbA1C levels. Mindfulness refers to moment-to-moment awareness. There are various mindfulness techniques, such as deep-breathing exercises, yoga, and meditation exercise.
- **By exercise.** In chapter 6, we discussed the importance of exercise in controlling blood glucose levels. However, studies have also shown that exercise reduces feelings of stress. Exercise is a great way to "blow off steam."
- **By seeking support.** Diabetes burnout is a real thing. One can seek support from a friend or family member. However, those who do not have diabetes might find it hard to relate. Therefore, one should consider joining online support groups through social media or joining in-person support groups. Again, seeking therapy from a medical professional is always an option.[23]
- **By staying organized.** Studies have shown that solid organizational practices are associated with lower chronic cortisol levels. Establishing a routine

will help one in managing diabetes. This includes scheduling time for meal preparation, cooking, blood glucose monitoring, exercising, and doctor's appointments.

- **By practicing good sleep hygiene.** In the previous chapter, we discussed the importance of sleep. We also discussed the concept of good sleep hygiene. One should aim for 7-9 hours of uninterrupted sleep per night.

We all experience stress. It would be somewhat untrue to say that one can eliminate all of the stress in one's life. Stress is inevitable. However, how one responds to stress and approaches stress is what makes all the difference.

In the next and final chapter, we will discuss cigarette smoking. We will explore some of the constituents which make up a cigarette and discover that cigarette smoke affects every system in the body.

We will also discuss nicotine withdrawal and what one can expect during the first five weeks of quitting smoking. We will also discuss some strategies that one can employ to help finally give up the habit.

10

IF YOU HAVEN'T ALREADY, NOW'S
THE TIME TO STOP SMOKING

In the previous chapter, we discussed the concept of stress and how it relates to hyperglycemia. We discovered that the WHO recognizes that "mental health is the foundation for the well-being and effective functioning of individuals."

We explored the three different types of stress; acute stress, episodic acute stress, and chronic stress. We learned about the physiology of acute stress and its impact on the body when it becomes chronic.

We also learned that acute stress is not necessarily "bad" and how in fact, it can be "good." We discussed an entity specific to diabetes which is known as "diabetes burnout."

We also discovered that stress manifests itself in many forms. Finally, we discussed how one with prediabetes or type 2 diabetes should approach stress.

This chapter will look at the negative impact of smoking on people with diabetes; cigarette smoking is a well-known risk factor for many diseases.

In fact, smoking is a *modifiable* risk factor for many chronic diseases such as cardiovascular disease, cancers, chronic obstructive lung disease, asthma, and diabetes.[1]

The keyword here is modifiable. Modifiable means that if one changes one's behavior (such as quitting smoking), one can decrease their risk of developing a disease or, in this case, diseases.

In order to fully grasp and understand the harmful effects of smoking, one must first have a basic understanding of exactly what smoking does to the body.

Conventionally, cigarette smoking is divided into two phases: a tar phase and a gas phase. The tar phase refers to the trapped material that accumulates when the smoke stream passes through the filter, known as particulate materials. And the gas phase refers to the gasses that pass through the filter.[2]

The tar phase consists of tiny particles, including water droplets, nicotine, and a collection of compounds, referred to as tar. Tar constitutes the primary source of carcinogenic compounds found in tobacco.

The gas-phase consists of carbon dioxide, carbon monoxide, ammonia, hydrogen cyanide, acetaldehyde, and acetone. Amongst these gases, carbon monoxide is the most toxic.[3]

During smoking, the complex biochemical mass of a cigarette is subjected to high temperatures and varying oxygen concentrations. The process of "lighting" a cigarette results in incomplete combustion that generates more than 7000 toxic compounds. And the main substances which constitute the gas phase, such as carbon monoxide and light aldehydes, immediately enter the lungs.

The compounds mainly found in the tar phase, such as nicotine, polycyclic aromatic compounds, nitrosamines, and heavy metals, are then absorbed through the skin, mucous membranes, alveoli, and the gastrointestinal system.[4]

It has been proven that chronic inhalation of cigarette smoke leads to altered cell proliferation, endothelial function, and immune response.[5] Therefore, cigarette smoking affects just about every organ in the body.

Let's take a look at some of the effects that cigarette smoking has on the body:

Hemoglobin is a protein in the red blood cells responsible for carrying oxygen from the lungs to the tissues and carbon dioxide from the tissues back to the lungs.

When carbon monoxide reacts with the hemoglobin in the blood, it forms what is known as carboxyhemoglobin.

Carboxyhemoglobin decreases the amount of oxygen delivered to the tissues. This lack of oxygen to the tissues causes an increase in blood pressure as the body tries to overcome tissue oxygenation.

The carbon dioxide and nicotine then increase the rate at which fatty materials are deposited in the arteries. This process is known as atherosclerosis which ultimately narrows the arteries. And narrowing the arteries leads to compromised and insufficient blood supply to the tissues and organs.[6]

Hence, a smoker is predisposed to atherosclerotic syndromes, including stable angina, acute coronary syndromes, sudden death, stroke, and abdominal aortic aneurysms.[7]

It has also been proven that carbon monoxide also leads to the hardening of the arteries. Furthermore, nicotine also causes the arteries to constrict, which increases the risk of blood clot formation and damages the arteries that supply the heart.[8]

Cigarette smoking has many adverse effects on the lungs and respiratory system. Another adverse effect is that tar accumulates in the lungs, which affects the functioning of the respiratory cilia. The respiratory cilia have a "sweeping" function and protect the lungs by "brushing out" unwanted particles and microbes. Due to the tar interfering with the normal functioning of the respiratory cilia, smokers are predisposed to developing bronchitis.

The toxic and harmful chemicals in cigarette smoke also alter the structure and function of the alveoli. Alveoli are the "air- sacs" found in the lungs which facilitate gaseous exchange in the lungs.

The destruction and altered function of the alveoli leads to a clinical entity known as emphysema. Those who suffer from emphysema are generally unable to participate in physical activities, and as the disease progresses, even mild physical exertion becomes problematic.

They suffer from breathlessness as their lungs can no longer perform an optimal gaseous exchange, whereby oxygen is taken up in the blood, and carbon dioxide is exhaled.

As mentioned earlier, tar constitutes the primary source of carcinogenic compounds found in tobacco, such as benzopyrene. More than 60 carcinogenic and mutagenic compounds have been identified in cigarette smoke.[9] Therefore, cigarette smokers are at a higher risk of developing lung cancers.

Cigarette smoking also aggravates asthma and predisposes one to pneumonia and pulmonary tuberculous due to the dysfunction that the chemicals found in cigarettes cause.[10]

Cigarette smoke has also been shown to have adverse effects on the gastrointestinal system.

The basis of this is that cigarette smoke induces the production of reactive oxygen species. It is the presence and action of antioxidants that neutralize the above-mentioned. If they are not balanced, this is when oxidative stress occurs, which results in tissue damage.

The effects that cigarette smoking causes on the gastrointestinal system are partially related to the large amounts of particulate materials ingested by the smoker. Also, the amount of nicotine in the gastric fluid is ten times higher than in the arterial blood and 80 times higher than in the venous blood.

It has also been suggested that chronic cigarette smoking can increase gastric acid secretion, thereby making the stomach acidic.

In addition, regular cigarette smoking has been shown to alter mucus production by the gastrointestinal mucosa and also causes dysfunction in mucosal repair. Cigarette smoke also has vasoconstrictor and procoagulant properties. And chronic cigarette smoke has been linked to peptic ulcers, inflammatory bowel disease, and gastric, esophageal, and colon cancer.[11]

Nicotine exerts its action principally on the brain's reward center. Some of the addictive properties are attributed to its ability to increase the synaptic neurotransmission of dopamine. Dopamine is involved in the rewarding effects of nicotine and therefore plays a vital role in the addictive properties of cigarette smoking. Dopamine is also responsible for creating a pleasurable sensation.[12]

Nicotine has also been shown to increase the levels of other neurotransmitters like acetylcholine. When one initially starts smoking cigarettes, acetylcholine signaling is increased. However, over time the brain begins to compensate for the increased signaling activity by decreasing the number of acetylcholine receptors. This is what causes what is known as nicotine tolerance. Therefore, more nicotine is needed to overcome this phenomenon.

Studies have shown that chronic cigarette smoking is also associated with cognitive decline and an increased risk of dementia. It has also been found that regular cigarette smoking is also associated with loss of brain volume.[13]

The association between nicotine and depression is also well established. A lifetime history of major depression is more than twice as common in smokers compared to non-smokers.

Nicotine is also associated with insomnia. This is because nicotine reduces sleep time, interferes with sleep initiation, and disrupts the sleep cycle.[14]

Cigarette smoking is also associated with erectile dysfunction. In addition, infants born to mothers who smoke during pregnancy are at a higher risk of intrauterine growth restriction.[15]

Calcium and vitamin D levels are also lower in those that smoke. In addition, cigarette smoking also reduces the ability of hormones such as estradiol in increasing bone mass. Hence, chronic cigarette smoking is also associated with osteoporosis.[16]

Lastly, smoking activates the hypothalamic-pituitary-adrenal axis, leading to increased production and secretion of hormones from the adrenal glands. These hormones include cortisol, adrenaline, and noradrenaline.

From the previous chapter, we know that these hormones increase one's heart rate and blood pressure. We also know that they are responsible for increasing one's blood glucose levels and mobilizing free fatty acids.[17]

So far, we have discussed the effects of cigarette smoke on the body in general. Next, we will discuss the relationship between cigarette smoking and type 2 diabetes.

A study conducted in Korea, which studied 4041 men over four years, found that past and current smokers were at an increased risk of developing type 2 diabetes. Another Japanese study also found that chronic cigarette smokers were also at a higher risk of developing diabetes. Furthermore, a British study also found that those who smoke cigarettes have a higher risk of developing diabetes.[18]

It has also been stated that cigarette smoke exposure worsens insulin resistance despite weight loss. This statement refers to both active and passive smoking. It must be noted that when we say insulin resistance is worsened with regard to cigarette smoke exposure, we mean in a dose-dependent manner.[19]

A study found that smoking reduced insulin-mediated glucose uptake by 10-40% in men who smoked than men who didn't smoke.

Specific to type 2 diabetes, a study found that in participants who smoked and who had type 2 diabetes, their insulin response to oral glucose was significantly higher than in non-smokers. Going back to the study, it was found that smoking induced insulin resistance, in a dose-dependent manner, in participants with type 2 diabetes and healthy participants.[20]

Smoking is also associated with increased visceral fat despite favorable changes in body mass index (BMI). From earlier chapters in this book, we discovered that increased fat in the liver and pancreas alters glucose metabolism.

We also learned that increased fat in the pancreas might induce dormancy of the B-cells of the pancreas; B-cells found in the pancreas are responsible for the production and secretion of insulin.[21]

Smoking is also associated with an increased incidence of non-alcoholic fatty liver disease (NAFLD) and non-alcoholic steatohepatitis (NASH).

These are two major causes of abnormal liver function. In addition, it interferes with the functioning of the liver, which includes glucose and fat metabolism, and further exacerbates insulin resistance.[22]

It must be noted here that the incidence of diabetes *may* be lower in those who smoke if smoking leads to weight loss and that weight loss leads to a decrease in visceral fat.

It must also be noted that with smoking cessation, the risk of developing diabetes decreases over time; however, it may paradoxically increase in association with weight gain, which tends to occur during the first 3-5 years following smoking cessation.[23]

Maternal smoking during pregnancy has also been linked to diabetes. This could be due to the damaging of the pancreatic B- cells in-utero.[24]

In those with established diabetes and those who use insulin, exposure to nicotine may increase the risk of profound hypoglycemia. This is thought to be because nicotine decreases the clearance of insulin from the body and enhances the action of insulin.[25]

A further point that helps prove that cigarette smoking causes insulin resistance is that the dyslipidemia (dyslipidemia refers to an abnormally high level of fats in the blood) found in insulin resistance mirrors that of the dyslipidemia found in those who smoke cigarettes. This is characterized by increased triglycerides and a reduction in high-density lipoprotein (HDL).[26]

Type 2 diabetes, if left untreated, is associated with many complications, including nephropathy, retinopathy, neuropathy, coronary heart disease, and stroke. And smoking is an independent risk factor for all of those mentioned above. And together, diabetes and cigarette smoking act synergistically in aggravating these complications.[27]

From all the above, it is understandable why the *Center for Disease Control and Prevention* (CDC) states that those who smoke are 30-40% more likely to develop diabetes than those who do not.

We have also discussed other complications of cigarette smoking which include inflammation due to the damage to tissues and cells, oxidative stress and cell damage, alterations in the functioning of the immune system, changes in lipid profiles, higher risk for developing respiratory conditions such as pneumonia and chronic obstructive pulmonary disease and increased risk of cardiovascular diseases such as heart attack and stroke.[28]

We have discussed how diabetes and smoking "act together" and can further worsen or bring about the onset of kidney and heart disease, eye diseases like retinopathy, which may ultimately lead to blindness, and accentuate nerve disease, leading to pain impairment in mobility.

In addition, cigarette smoking and diabetes both cause alterations in immunity and a reduction in blood flow. These compounding effects accentuate the occurrence of infections, ulcers, and the formation of blood clots.[29] And of course, smoking is also associated with many other types of cancers.

Unfortunately, many of the combined health effects of cigarette smoking and diabetes make it even more difficult to make healthier lifestyle choices. For instance, the combination of cardiovascular disease, nerve damage, and reduced lung function can make it harder for one to exercise.[30]

There is no safe way to smoke. The best way to lower one's risks from smoking is to quit or to at least drastically cut down.[31]

Unfortunately, 50% of smokers die from a smoking-related disease. Furthermore, the life expectancy of one in four smokers is reduced by as much as 15-20 years.[32]

The following strategies may help lower the risks associated with cigarette smoking and diabetes:

- **Healthy eating:** Throughout chapters 1-4, we discussed different approaches to healthy eating as well as the place of intermittent fasting in controlling and potentially achieving remission from prediabetes and type 2 diabetes. We now know that eating a diet rich in fruits and vegetables and whole grains and avoiding processed foods, sugar, and simple carbohydrates lowers the risk of cardiovascular disease.[33]
- **Exercise and physical activity:** In chapter 6, we discussed the importance of exercise. We discovered that exercise supports glucose

metabolism, and when combined with healthy eating, reduces the chance of obesity.[34]

- **Following the treatment plan:** In those with hard-to-control diabetes, it is essential that they follow their prescribed treatment plan. Controlling one's diabetes is the only way to mitigate complications.[35]
- **Quitting smoking:** Or at least drastically cutting back. Stopping smoking reduces the future risk of tobacco-related diseases and improves life expectancy by about ten years.[36]

Quitting smoking may seem like a tedious and strenuous task. Ultimately, the rewards outweigh this-and they occur almost immediately.

Within 24-hours of quitting smoking, one's heart rate, blood pressure, and peripheral circulation begin to improve. By the end of the first day, the carbon monoxide levels in one's lungs decrease to normal levels. Within 48-72 hours, all of the nicotine has left the body. At this stage, one's taste and smell are on their way to recovering. After 1-3 months, one's lung function may have improved by as much as 30%. At about six months, shortness of breath has significantly improved. One year after quitting smoking, one's risk of a heart attack decreases to half that of a smoker's risk. After ten years, the risk of lung cancer reduces by 50-60%. And after 15 years, the risk of heart attack and stroke falls to the levels of someone who has never smoked.[37]

It is important to be aware that one is highly likely to experience nicotine withdrawal after quitting smoking. Nicotine withdrawal involves physical, mental, and emotional symptoms.

It is said that the first week, especially days 3 through 5, are always the worst. This is because all the nicotine has now cleared out of one's body. At this stage, one may start experiencing cravings, headaches, fatigue, constipation, and insomnia.

Soon after this, one may start experiencing mental symptoms of nicotine withdrawal which include anxiety, depression, and irritability. However, these will begin to taper off after a few weeks.

Here's a timeline of what one can expect[38]:

- **Thirty minutes-4 hours:** the effects of nicotine will begin to wear off, and one will start to crave another cigarette.
- **Ten hours:** one may feel restless and start physically craving a cigarette. At this time, it is not unusual for one to experience feelings of sadness and hopelessness.
- **Twenty-four hours:** one may start to become irritable, and one's appetite may increase.
- **Two days:** as the nicotine starts to clear out of one's body, one may begin to experience headaches.
- **Three days:** at this stage, all the nicotine should be cleared out of one's body. After that, one's cravings

for a cigarette may taper off, but anxiety will start
to rise.

- **2-4 weeks:** one's appetite will begin to normalize,
  and the brain fog will start clearing up. Depression
  and anxiety will begin alleviating.
- **Five weeks:** from here on, one must keep a solid
  mental hold.

Now that one is aware of what one can expect to
experience over the first four weeks of quitting smoking;
one needs to have some strategies to overcome the urge to
smoke:[39]

- **Cold turkey.** Research has shown that those who
  quit "cold turkey" are more likely to be successful
  than those who quit gradually
- **Don't give up.** Many people attempt to quit
  smoking several times before they do. It's not a
  failure. One can always learn from the experience
  and "try again next time."
- **Recognize the addiction.** Withdrawal from
  nicotine is uncomfortable and, at times, difficult to
  bear. Recognize it for what it is-the body
  withdrawing from a substance. The symptoms
  won't last forever
- **Break the habit.** Find new and healthy habits. One
  should try and change their behavior around
  smoking. For example, if the first thing one does in
  the morning is have a cigarette, perhaps one
  should consider going for a walk instead

- **Ask about nicotine replacement therapy and quit assistance medication.** However, before starting this endeavor, one should consult with one's doctor
- **Counseling.** This may help one understand why one thinks smoking helps one cope. Counseling may also provide emotional support and understanding during nicotine withdrawal
- **Unity.** Convince others to join. This helps with motivation and encouragement

We all know that smoking is harmful and, other than a "perceived" coping mechanism, has absolutely no benefits to health-let alone in those with prediabetes and type 2 diabetes.

Thank You!

Customer reviews

⭐⭐⭐⭐⭐ **5 out of 5** ⌄

14 customer ratings

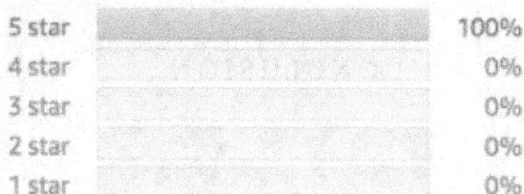

5 star	████████████	100%
4 star		0%
3 star		0%
2 star		0%
1 star		0%

Review this product

Share your thoughts with other customers

> Write a customer review

I would be incredibly thankful if you could take just 60 seconds to write a brief review on Amazon. Even if it's just a few sentences, it will help me and others like you!

CONCLUSION

I n conclusion, we should look to what the great French philosopher Voltaire once said; "The art of medicine consists in amusing the patient while nature cures the disease."

With regards to this book, we define "nature" as following a lifestyle in which one prioritizes a healthy and nutritious diet, changes one's behavior towards food, decreases visceral fat, exercises regularly, favors water over other beverages, practices good sleep hygiene, prioritizes mental health and quits cigarette smoking.

Voltaire lived between 1694 and 1778. We are now in the 21st century, and medicine has come a long way.

Throughout this book, we have stressed the importance of seeking advice from a medical practitioner before incorporating any lifestyle changes.

Voltaire lived in an era where science was just not what it is today. There were limited medications and treatment options available. It must be stressed that one is not a "failure" if one cannot control their diabetes with lifestyle changes alone.

The phrase "everybody is different" is quite literal. The human body adapts and changes according to genetics, medications, and lifestyle. What may work for Sam may not work for Sally.

The point is that the lifestyle changes we have proposed are not unreasonable or particularly difficult and are backed by science. So why not give it a go? Of course, under medical supervision.

We acknowledge that, well, quite frankly, all of this information is quite challenging too, for lack of a better word, "digest." Therefore, it only fits that we conclude all of this material in an easily digestible manner.

In chapter 1, we defined prediabetes and type 2 diabetes. We learned that prediabetes refers to a condition whereby blood sugar levels are higher than what they should be but not high enough to be classified as type 2 diabetes.

We also learned that prediabetes consists of two clinical entities; impaired fasting glucose (IFG) and impaired glucose tolerance (IGT). We also looked at how normoglycemia, prediabetes, and diabetes are defined.

Result	Fasting blood glucose	Random blood glucose	A1C test	Oral glucose tolerance test
Normoglycemia	< 99mg/dL (5.49mmol/L)	N/A	Below 5.7%	< 140mg/dL (7.77mmol/L)
Prediabetes	100-125mg/dL (5.55-6.94mmol/L)	N/A	5.7-6.4%	140-199mg/dL (7.77-11.04mmol/L)
Diabetes	>126mg/dL (6.99mmol/L)	> 200mg/dL (11.1mmol/L)	> 6.5%	> 200mg/dL (11.1mmol/L)

Table 1: showing the results of diagnostic tests for normoglycemia, prediabetes, and diabetes.

We discovered what insulin resistance is. Insulin resistance is synonymous with prediabetes. Body tissues, especially the muscles, become resistant to the effects of insulin. This results in less glucose being taken up by the body tissues, ultimately leading to a high glucose concentration in the blood.

This also leads to the pancreas going into a state of "overdrive." Ultimately, we learned that there is a relative insulin deficiency in prediabetes rather than an absolute insulin deficiency. However, we also learned that if the above process is allowed to continue, it will result in type 2 diabetes.

We then went on to define type 2 diabetes. And explained that type 2 diabetes is characterized by variable degrees of insulin resistance, impaired insulin secretion, and excessive glucose production by the liver.

We also discussed the risk factors for type 2 diabetes which included being overweight, being 45 years of age and older, having a first degree relative with type 2 diabetes, having an inactive lifestyle, having a previous history of gestational diabetes (pregnancy-induced diabetes), having polycystic ovarian syndrome, being of African American, Hispanic/Latino American, American Indian, or Pacific Islander descent, having prediabetes, and having non-alcoholic fatty liver disease.

We then went on to discuss the complications of type 2 diabetes. These included coronary heart disease, stroke, peripheral vascular disease, diabetic neuropathy, diabetic retinopathy, and diabetic nephropathy. We concluded that having tight control of diabetes decreased the chances of developing complications.

We went on to find out that research has shown that there are huge health benefits associated with just losing 5% of your total body weight. At this point, we discussed the concept of body mass index (BMI) and discussed that although a widely used tool, it is not that accurate as it does not account for visceral fat. We then went on to discuss the concept of "metabolically obese normal weight" (MONW).

In chapter 2, we started embracing the topic of diet and its importance. We explained that the aim of cultivating a clean and healthy diet is to help restore normal blood glucose levels.

First, we discussed the fundamentals of "eating clean" and learned about the NOVA groups for food processing which classifies processed foods into four groups.

After delving into the classification of processed foods, we discussed that fundamentally clean eating is prioritizing group 1 and group 2 processed foods, minimizing one's intake of group 3 processed food products, and avoiding group 4 processed foods. We went further and then discussed the principles of clean eating.

We then defined what a balanced diet is and discussed the different food groups and the importance of each food group. We then went on to discuss the "ChooseMyPlate" initiative, which recommended filling half of one's plate with fruits and vegetables, filling just over one quarter with grains, filling just under one quarter with protein-containing foods, and adding a dairy or a non-dairy substitute on the side.

Finally, we went on to discuss the importance and concepts of the glycemic index and glycemic load.

We explained that the glycemic index accounts for how different carbohydrate-rich foods directly affect blood glucose levels. And the glycemic load helps establish how different sized portions of different foods compare in terms of their blood glucose-raising effect.

In chapter 3, we delved further into diet and discussed "cutting carbs the right way." We discovered that carbohydrates were the nutrient that had the greatest effect in raising blood glucose levels and required the most insulin for metabolism.

We further found that different carbohydrates affected individuals differently based on genetics and an individual's baseline insulin sensitivity.

We also looked at grams of digestible carbohydrates per portion size with regards to different fruits. We discovered that not all fruits were equal when it came to their carbohydrate content.

Throughout chapter 4, we discussed intermittent fasting. We discovered that intermittent fasting is not a "diet fad" and that our ancestors have been practicing intermittent fasting for centuries.

We found that intermittent fasting is based on the principle of consuming very little to no calories for periods ranging from 12 hours to several days with a regular pattern.

We explored three different approaches to intermittent fasting; the 5:2 plan, the 24-hour plan, and the time-restricted plan.

We stressed that one should choose a method which suits their lifestyle best. We explained that the principle of intermittent fasting is based on the fact that if the body does not receive an immediate energy source, insulin levels will decrease. The body will then use its stored potential energy, which is found in fat, for an immediate energy source. And during this time, the fat cells will release free fatty acids and glycerol. Hence, fat is "burned off." However, for this to be facilitated, insulin levels must decrease low enough and for a long enough period of time.

We concluded by mentioning the importance of eating healthy and nutritious foods, especially when fasting, as the body always needs energy. We stated that the key to remember when it comes to intermittent fasting is that after 24-hours of fasting, the body will no longer use fat as its energy source. Instead, the body will use proteins as its energy source.

One needs to remember that proteins play an integral role in maintaining various structural and metabolic functions. Therefore, one should not fast beyond 24-hours, and we mentioned that intermittent fasting does not mean "dry fasting." One is allowed to consume calorie-free beverages such as unsweetened coffee, tea, and water.

It was only in chapter 5 that we discussed the importance of weight loss. Throughout chapters 2-4, we discussed different dietary strategies but did not emphasize weight loss itself. Hence, we dedicated a whole chapter to it.

We learned that weight loss could help achieve remission from prediabetes and type 2 diabetes. We discovered that weight loss facilitated better pancreatic B-cell functioning. This is because better B-cell functioning is associated with reducing both liver and pancreatic fat.

We also mentioned that it had been postulated that excessive fat in the liver and pancreas might induce a state of "dormancy" within the pancreatic B-cells. However, it must also be noted that there may be a "personal fat threshold" and that, therefore, one individual might have to lose more weight than the person sitting next to them to achieve remission.

We also looked at a study that showed that one's likelihood of achieving remission from diabetes was more likely in the first five years after being diagnosed. However, we also mentioned that this does not mean that they will not achieve remission if one has long-standing type 2 diabetes. It just means that they are less likely.

In chapter 6, we discussed exercise. We returned to chapter 5 and learned that exercise along with a healthy diet helped aid in decreasing the fat content of the liver and the pancreas. Hence, exercise and diet go hand-in-hand.

We also discovered that exercise improved insulin sensitivity. When muscles are active, which occurs during physical activity and exercise, they use glucose as their primary energy source. The use of glucose as a primary source of energy prevents the accumulation of glucose in the blood-instead of glucose staying in the blood, the muscles then took up the glucose.

We explained that exercise resulted in an immediate increase in insulin sensitivity. And that this increase in insulin sensitivity lasted between 2-48 hours, depending on the type of exercise.

We also discussed aerobic and anaerobic exercises in detail. And we looked to the American Diabetes Association and what they recommended when it came to physical activity and type 2 diabetes; they recommended:

- Exercising daily, or at least not allowing more than two days to pass between exercise sessions, this was recommended to enhance insulin action.
- For optimal glycemic and health outcomes, adults with type 2 diabetes should participate in both aerobic and anaerobic exercises.
- To prevent or delay the onset of type 2 diabetes in those that are at a higher risk of developing type 2 diabetes or have already established prediabetes, one should participate in at least 150 minutes of exercise per week and incorporate dietary changes which should aim to result in weight loss of 5-7%.

In chapter 7, we discussed the importance of hydration. We learned that water intake is derived from two primary sources; directly through drinking fluids and indirectly through eating food substances with high water content, such as certain fruits and vegetables.

We discussed the functions of water which included aiding in the digestion, absorption, and transport of other nutrients, helping maintain the structural and functional integrity of the cells, aiding in the removal of waste products and toxins, acting as a medium for biochemical reactions, aiding in thermoregulation and helping in maintaining lubrication of cavities and joints.

New evidence suggested that bodily fluids may also have a significant role in hormone release, cell proliferation, and even cell death.

We discussed the concept of dehydration and its effects on the body. We discovered that increased water intake was associated with lower blood glucose levels. This is partly because vasopressin acts not only on the kidneys but also on the liver.

We explained that vasopressin is the hormone that is released when the body needs to conserve water. However, it also acts on the liver and encourages the release of glucose from the liver into the blood.

We also discovered that dehydration led to glucose in the blood becoming more concentrated. We then went on to find that hyperglycemia led to polyuria which further aggravated water loss. We then discussed alcohol and why it should be limited in those with prediabetes and type 2 diabetes.

We then concluded by saying that according to the American Diabetes Association, a diabetic's daily water intake requirement is the same as that of a healthy person unless otherwise specified by a personal physician.

The Institute of Medicine suggested that women should drink about 2.2 liters of fluid per day, and men should drink about 3 liters of fluid per day.

In chapter 8, we discussed sleep. We discovered that sleep is rather complicated. We further discussed the different theories around sleep; inactive theory, energy conservative theory, restorative theory, and brain plasticity theory.

We concluded that the importance and function of sleep are not based on one theory alone but rather a combination of all of these theories.

We discussed some of the areas in the brain which facilitate sleep. We further discussed the two phases of sleep; rapid eye movement (REM) and non-rapid eye movement (NREM).

We discussed a review that revealed that difficulty in initiating sleep increased the risk of developing type 2 diabetes by 55%, while difficulty maintaining sleep increased its risk by 74%.

We explored how good sleep hygiene aided in better control of prediabetes and type 2 diabetes. Ultimately, we discovered that poor sleep led to disturbances in the neuroendocrine axis, which led to weight gain and perhaps even insulin resistance.

In chapter 9, we broached the subject of mental health. First, we discussed stress and how different individuals perceived and manifested stress differently.

We mentioned that the American Psychological Association recognized three forms of stress; acute stress, episodic acute stress, and chronic stress.

Next, we discussed the acute stress response and the different hormones involved. We concluded by stating that acute stress was not necessarily bad and that acute stress is an evolutionary protective mechanism.

We then explored chronic stress and discovered that when the acute stress mechanism was allowed to continue, it had adverse effects on just about every system of the body. Ultimately, we concluded by saying that chronic stress disrupted the neuroendocrine axis, leading to hormonal changes that ultimately affected blood glucose levels.

And finally, in chapter 10, we discussed cigarette smoking. We briefly touched on the constituents of a cigarette and discovered that the process of "lighting" a cigarette resulted in incomplete combustion that generated more than 7000 toxic compounds.

We discussed the adverse effects of cigarette smoking and stated that cigarette smoke affected every system in the body.

We looked at several studies which showed that cigarette smoking placed one at a higher risk of developing type 2 diabetes.

We stated that the complications of cigarette smoking and type 2 diabetes could synergistically worsen each other's complications.

We discussed nicotine withdrawal and what one should expect over the first five weeks of stopping smoking.

And finally, we concluded by saying that there was simply no safe way to smoke.

Prediabetes and type 2 diabetes is a complex clinical entity. Type 2 diabetes is a disorder of the endocrine system. And the endocrine system is responsible for the production and secretion of hormones.

Ultimately, this book is about implementing strategies that help "normalize" the endocrine system.

In essence, one can help control or perhaps even achieve remission from prediabetes and type 2 diabetes if one simply incorporates strategies into their daily life to harmonize one's hormones.

The human body is robust and yet delicate. Like water and fire, the human body is a great servant but a bad master.

If I can reverse mine, then so can you! ☺

Especially

For You

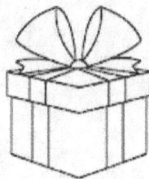

As a thank you, grab your <u>Free</u> Copy of "99 ways to lose 1 Pound Every Month While Still Eating The Foods You Love" and start your journey to remission today!

Visit the link below and enjoy

www.jonahyjoseph.com/Resources

RESOURCES

MY STORY

1. https://www.webmd.com/cold-and-flu/ss/slideshow-how-you-suppress-immune-system
2. https://www.jonahyjoseph.com/My-Story
3. https://patient.info/allergies-blood-immune/immune-system-diseases/immune-suppression
   https://www.jonahyjoseph.com/ My-Story

1. UNDERSTANDING YOUR CONDITION

1. Prediabetes - Your Chance to Prevent Type 2 Diabetes. (2020, June 11). Retrieved from Centers for Disease Control and Prevention: www.cdc.gov/diabetes/basics/prediabetes.html
2. Longo, D., Fauci, A., & Kasper, D; et al (2013). Endocrinology and Metabolism. In Harrison's Manual of Medicine (p. 1138). McGraw-Hill.   https://archive.org/details/HarrisonsManualOfMedicine19thEd/page/n921/mode/2up?q=impaired+fasting+glucose
3. World Health Organization. (2021). Retrieved from Obesity and Overweight: https://www.who.int/news-room/fact-sheets/detail/obesity-and-overweight
4. Mayo Clinic. (2020, October 3). Retrieved from Polycystic ovarian syndrome (PCOS): https://www.mayoclinic.org/diseases-conditions/pcos/symptoms-causes/syc-20353439
5. Prediabetes - Your Chance to Prevent Type 2 Diabetes. (2020, June 11). Retrieved from Centers for Disease Control and Prevention: https://www.cdc.gov/diabetes/basics/prediabetes.html
6. Tests for Type 1 Diabetes, Type 2 Diabetes, and Prediabetes. (2019, May 15). Retrieved from Centers for Disease Control and Prevention: https://www.cdc.gov/diabetes/basics/getting-tested.html

7. Tests for Type 1 Diabetes, Type 2 Diabetes, and Prediabetes. (2019, May 15). Retrieved from Centers for Disease Control and Prevention:
   https://www.cdc.gov/diabetes/basics/getting-tested.html

8. Davidson, S; Walker, BR; College, BR; et al. (2014). Diabetes Mellitus. Davidson's Principals and Practice of Medicine (p. 805). Elsevier; JCI - MAPK phosphatase–3 promotes hepatic gluconeogenesis: www.jci.org/articles/view/43250
   Insulin resistance: what it is and how to prevent it: www.diabetescarecommunity.ca/diabetes-overview-articles/insulin-resistance-what-it-is-and-how-to-prevent-it

9. The University of Pittsburgh. (2021). Retrieved from Diabetes Prevention Support Center: https://www.diabetesprevention.pitt.edu/for-the-public/diabetes-prevention-program-dpp/

10. Harvard Health Publishing Harvard Medical School. (2018, September 5). Retrieved from Healthy lifestyle can prevent diabetes (and even reverse it): https://www.health.harvard.edu/blog/healthy-lifestyle-can-prevent-diabetes-and-even-reverse-it-2018090514698

11. Longo, D., Fauci, A., & Kasper, D; et al (2013). Endocrinology and Metabolism. In Harrison's Manual of Medicine (p. 1138). McGraw-Hill.
    https://archive.org/details/HarrisonsManualOfMedicine19thEd/page/n921/mode/2up?q=impaired+fasting+glucose

12. Davidson, S; Walker, BR; College, BR; et al. (2014). Diabetes Mellitus. Davidson's Principals and Practice of Medicine (p. 805). Elsevier; JCI - MAPK phosphatase–3 promotes hepatic gluconeogenesis: www.jci.org/articles/view/43250
    Insulin resistance: what it is and how to prevent it: www.diabetescarecommunity.ca/diabetes-overview-articles/insulin-resistance-what-it-is-and-how-to-prevent-it/

13. Tests for Type 1 Diabetes, Type 2 Diabetes, and Prediabetes. (2019, May 15). Retrieved from Centers for Disease Control and Prevention:
    https://www.cdc.gov/diabetes/basics/getting-tested.html

14. Centers for Disease Control and Prevention. (2020, March 24). Retrieved from Diabetes symptoms: https://www.cdc.gov/diabetes/basics/symptoms.html

Diet Tips for Diabetes Patients | nurishingly.com. https://www. nurishingly.com/diet/diet-tips-for-diabetes-patients/

15. Centers for Disease Control and Prevention. (2020, March 24). Retrieved from Diabetes risk factors: https://www.cdc.gov/ diabetes/basics/risk-factors.html

16. Longo, D., Fauci, A., & Kasper, D; et al (2013). Endocrinology and Metabolism. In Harrison's Manual of Medicine (p. 1138). McGraw-Hill.
    https://archive.org/details/HarrisonsManualOfMedi-cine19thEd/page/n921/mode/2up?q=impaired+fasting+glucose

17. http://www.imed.ro/forum/viewtopic.php?t=1043

18. http://www.imed.ro/forum/viewtopic.php?t=1043

19. http://www.imed.ro/forum/viewtopic.php?t=1043

20. http://www.imed.ro/forum/viewtopic.php?t=1043

21. http://www.imed.ro/forum/viewtopic.php?t=1043

22. http://www.imed.ro/forum/viewtopic.php?t=1043

23. http://www.imed.ro/forum/viewtopic.php?t=1043

24. Diabetes UK. (n.d.). Retrieved from Reversing Type 2 Diabetes: https://www.diabetes.org.uk/diabetes-the-basics/type-2-reverse

25. Nursing Times. (2015, March 16). Retrieved from Reversing Type 2 Diabetes with Lifestyle Changes: https:// https://www. nursingtimes.net/clinical-archive/diabetes-clinical-archive/ reversing-type-2-diabetes-with-lifestyle-change-16-03-2015/

26. Diabetes UK. (n.d.). Retrieved from Reversing Type 2 Diabetes: https://www.diabetes.org.uk/diabetes-the-basics/type-2-reverse

27. Centers for Disease Control and Prevention. (2021, March 3). Retrieved from Defining Adult Overweight and Obesity: https:// www.cdc.gov/obesity/adult/defining.html

28. Ding, C., Chan, Z., & Magkos, F. (2016). Lean, but not healthy: the 'metabolically obese, normal-weight phenotype. Current Opinion in Clinical Nutrition and Metabolic Care, 408-417. https://doi.org/10. 1097/MCO.0000000000000317

2. DIET PART ONE: CULTIVATE A CLEAN
AND HEALTHY DIET

1. Higuera, V. (2020, June 5). Healthline. Retrieved from 8 Lifestyle Tips to Help Reverse Prediabetes Naturally: www.healthline.com/health/diabetes/how-to-reverse-prediabetes-naturally
2. Higuera, V. (2020, June 5). Healthline. Retrieved from 8 Lifestyle Tips to Help Reverse Prediabetes Naturally: www.healthline.com/health/diabetes/how-to-reverse-prediabetes-naturally
3. Brown, E. (2020, August 14). Mayo Clinic- Healthy Lifestyle. Nutrition and Healthy Eating. Retrieved from What does it mean to eat clean? https://www.mayoclinic.org/healthy-lifestyle/nutrition-and-healthy-eating/in-depth/what-does-it-mean-to-eat-clean/art-20270125
   3 Ways to Reduce Blood Sugar - wikiHow. https://www.wikihow.com/Reduce-Blood-Sugar
4. Harguth, A. (2017, January 3). Mayo Clinic. Retrieved from Processed foods: What you should know: https://www.mayoclinichealthsystem.org/hometown-health/speaking-of-health/processed-foods-what-you-should-know
5. Brown, E. (2020, August 14). Mayo Clinic- Healthy Lifestyle. Nutrition and Healthy Eating. Retrieved from What does it mean to eat clean?: https://www.mayoclinic.org/healthy-lifestyle/nutrition-and-healthy-eating/in-depth/what-does-it-mean-to-eat-clean/art-20270125
   3 Ways to Reduce Blood Sugar - wikiHow. https://www.wikihow.com/Reduce-Blood-Sugar
6. Brown, E. (2020, August 14). Mayo Clinic- Healthy Lifestyle. Nutrition and Healthy Eating. Retrieved from What does it mean to eat clean?: https://www.mayoclinic.org/healthy-lifestyle/nutrition-and-healthy-eating/in-depth/what-does-it-mean-to-eat-clean/art-20270125
   3 Ways to Reduce Blood Sugar - wikiHow. https://www.wikihow.com/Reduce-Blood-Sugar
7. Brown, E. (2020, August 14). Mayo Clinic- Healthy Lifestyle. Nutrition and Healthy Eating. Retrieved from What does it mean to eat clean?: https://www.mayoclinic.org/healthy-lifestyle/

nutrition-and-healthy-eating/in-depth/what-does-it-mean-to-eat-clean/art-20270125

3 Ways to Reduce Blood Sugar - wikiHow. https://www.wikihow.com/Reduce-Blood-Sugar

8. Open Food Facts. (n.d.). Retrieved from Nova groups for food processing: https://world.openfoodfacts.org/nova#:~:text=Processed%20foods%2C%20such%20as%20bottled%20vegetables%2C%20canned%20fish%2C

9. Brown, E. (2020, August 14). Mayo Clinic- Healthy Lifestyle. Nutrition and Healthy Eating. Retrieved from What does it mean to eat clean?: https://www.mayoclinic.org/healthy-lifestyle/nutrition-and-healthy-eating/in-depth/what-does-it-mean-to-eat-clean/art-20270125

3 Ways to Reduce Blood Sugar - wikiHow. https://www.wikihow.com/Reduce-Blood-Sugar

10. Spritzler, F. (2019, April 8). Healthline. Retrieved from 11 Simple Ways to Start Clean Eating Today: www.healthline.com/nutrition/11-ways-to-eat-clean#TOC_TITLE_HDR_3

11. Spritzler, F. (2019, April 8). Healthline. Retrieved from 11 Simple Ways to Start Clean Eating Today: www.healthline.com/nutrition/11-ways-to-eat-clean#TOC_TITLE_HDR_3

Cleveland Clinic. (2019, December 11). Retrieved from What to Eat If You've Been Diagnosed with Prediabetes: https://health.clevelandclinic.org/what-to-eat-if-youve-been-diagnosed-with-prediabetes/

12. Spritzler, F. (2019, April 8). Healthline. Retrieved from 11 Simple Ways to Start Clean Eating Today: www.healthline.com/nutrition/11-ways-to-eat-clean#TOC_TITLE_HDR_3

13. Spritzler, F. (2019, April 8). Healthline. Retrieved from 11 Simple Ways to Start Clean Eating Today: www.healthline.com/nutrition/11-ways-to-eat-clean#TOC_TITLE_HDR_3

14. Cleveland Clinic. (2019, December 11). Retrieved from What to Eat If You've Been Diagnosed With Prediabetes: https://health.clevelandclinic.org/what-to-eat-if-youve-been-diagnosed-with-prediabetes/

15. Spritzler, F. (2019, April 8). Healthline. Retrieved from 11 Simple Ways to Start Clean Eating Today: www.healthline.com/nutrition/11-ways-to-eat-clean#TOC_TITLE_HDR_3

16. Cleveland Clinic. (2019, December 11). Retrieved from What to Eat If You've Been Diagnosed With Prediabetes: https://health. clevelandclinic.org/what-to-eat-if-youve-been-diagnosed-with-prediabetes/

17. Cleveland Clinic. (2019, December 11). Retrieved from What to Eat If You've Been Diagnosed With Prediabetes: https://health. clevelandclinic.org/what-to-eat-if-youve-been-diagnosed-with-prediabetes/
Spritzler, F. (2019, April 8). Healthline. Retrieved from 11 Simple Ways to Start Clean Eating Today: www.healthline.com/nutrition/ 11-ways-to-eat-clean#TOC_TITLE_HDR_3

18. Spritzler, F. (2019, April 8). Healthline. Retrieved from 11 Simple Ways to Start Clean Eating Today: www.healthline.com/nutrition/ 11-ways-to-eat-clean#TOC_TITLE_HDR_3

19. Spritzler, F. (2019, April 8). Healthline. Retrieved from 11 Simple Ways to Start Clean Eating Today: www.healthline.com/nutrition/ 11-ways-to-eat-clean#TOC_TITLE_HDR_3

20. Spritzler, F. (2019, April 8). Healthline. Retrieved from 11 Simple Ways to Start Clean Eating Today: www.healthline.com/nutrition/ 11-ways-to-eat-clean#TOC_TITLE_HDR_3

21. Spritzler, F. (2019, April 8). Healthline. Retrieved from 11 Simple Ways to Start Clean Eating Today: www.healthline.com/nutrition/ 11-ways-to-eat-clean#TOC_TITLE_HDR_3

22. Spritzler, F. (2019, April 8). Healthline. Retrieved from 11 Simple Ways to Start Clean Eating Today: www.healthline.com/nutrition/ 11-ways-to-eat-clean#TOC_TITLE_HDR_3

23. The Free Dictionary by Farlex. (n.d.). Retrieved from Balanced Diet: https://medical-dictionary.thefreedictionary.com/ balanced+diet

24. Krans, B. (2020, June 29). Healthline. Retrieved from Balanced Diet: https://www.healthline.com/health/balanced-diet#what-to-eat

25. Krans, B. (2020, June 29). Healthline. Retrieved from Balanced Diet: https://www.healthline.com/health/balanced-diet#what-to-eat

26. Frothingham. (2019, March 7). Healthline. Retrieved from What You Should Know About Fruit for a Diabetes Diet: https://www. healthline.com/health/fruits-for-diabetes

27. Diet Health Club. (2014, January 16). Retrieved from Benefits of Low Fat Dairy Products: http://www.diethealthclub.com/ therapeutic-value-of-different-foods/low-fat-dairy.html

Bergtholdt, S. (n.d.). Livestrong.com. Retrieved from The Functions of the Six Major Food Groups: https://www.livestrong.com/article/382946-the-functions-of-the-six-major-food-groups/

28. Diet Health Club. (2014, January 16). Retrieved from Benefits of Low Fat Dairy Products: http://www.diethealthclub.com/therapeutic-value-of-different-foods/low-fat-dairy.html

Bergtholdt, S. (n.d.). Livestrong.com. Retrieved from The Functions of the Six Major Food Groups: https://www.livestrong.com/article/382946-the-functions-of-the-six-major-food-groups/

29. Diet Health Club. (2014, January 16). Retrieved from Benefits of Low Fat Dairy Products: http://www.diethealthclub.com/therapeutic-value-of-different-foods/low-fat-dairy.html

Bergtholdt, S. (n.d.). Livestrong.com. Retrieved from The Functions of the Six Major Food Groups: https://www.livestrong.com/article/382946-the-functions-of-the-six-major-food-groups/

Busch, S. (2018, December 7). SFGate. Retrieved from Does Protein Have Vitamins?: https://healthyeating.sfgate.com/protein-vitamins-10756.html

30. Bergtholdt, S. (n.d.). Livestrong.com. Retrieved from The Functions of the Six Major Food Groups: https://www.livestrong.com/article/382946-the-functions-of-the-six-major-food-groups/

31. Krans, B. (2020, June 29). Healthline. Retrieved from Balanced Diet: https://www.healthline.com/health/balanced-diet#what-to-eat

32. Krans, B. (2020, June 29). Healthline. Retrieved from Balanced Diet: https://www.healthline.com/health/balanced-diet#what-to-eat

33. Van De Walle, G. (2018, June 20). Healthline. Retrieved from 9 Important Functions of Protein in Your Body: www.healthline.com/nutrition/functions-of-protein#TOC_TITLE_HDR_2

34. Hite, A. (2021, February 11). Diet Doctor. Retrieved from How to Reverse Your Type 2 Diabetes: https://www.dietdoctor.com/diabetes

Understanding the glycemic index and how to use it: https://www.wellbeing.com.au/body/health/gi-know-how.html

35. Harvard TH Chan School of Public Health- The Nutrition Source. (n.d.). Retrieved from Carbohydrates and Blood Sugar: www.hsph.harvard.edu/nutritionsource/carbohydrates/carbohydrates-and-blood-sugar/

36. Hite, A. (2021, February 11). Diet Doctor. Retrieved from How to Reverse Your Type 2 Diabetes: https://www.dietdoctor.com/diabetes Understanding the glycemic index and how to use it: https://www.wellbeing.com.au/body/health/gi-know-how.html

37. Harvard TH Chan School of Public Health- The Nutrition Source. (n.d.). Retrieved from Carbohydrates and Blood Sugar: www.hsph.harvard.edu/nutritionsource/carbohydrates/carbohydrates-and-blood-sugar/

38. Harvard TH Chan School of Public Health- The Nutrition Source. (n.d.). Retrieved from Carbohydrates and Blood Sugar: www.hsph.harvard.edu/nutritionsource/carbohydrates/carbohydrates-and-blood-sugar/

39. Harvard TH Chan School of Public Health- The Nutrition Source. (n.d.). Retrieved from Carbohydrates and Blood Sugar: www.hsph.harvard.edu/nutritionsource/carbohydrates/carbohydrates-and-blood-sugar/

40. Brown, E. (2020, August 14). Mayo Clinic- Healthy Lifestyle. Nutrition and Healthy Eating. Retrieved from What does it mean to eat clean?: https://www.mayoclinic.org/healthy-lifestyle/nutrition-and-healthy-eating/in-depth/what-does-it-mean-to-eat-clean/art-20270125

41. Brown, E. (2020, August 14). Mayo Clinic- Healthy Lifestyle. Nutrition and Healthy Eating. Retrieved from What does it mean to eat clean?: https://www.mayoclinic.org/healthy-lifestyle/nutrition-and-healthy-eating/in-depth/what-does-it-mean-to-eat-clean/art-20270125

42. Fiona S. Atkinson, RD, Kaye Foster-Powell, RD and Jennie C. Brand-Miller, PHD. (2008, December 31). American Diabetes Association. Retrieved from International Tables of Glycemic Index and Glycemic Load Values 2008: https://care.diabetesjournals.org/content/31/12/2281

43. Fiona S. Atkinson, RD, Kaye Foster-Powell, RD and Jennie C. Brand-Miller, PHD. (2008, December 31). American Diabetes Association. Retrieved from International Tables of Glycemic Index and Glycemic Load Values 2008: https://care.diabetesjournals.org/content/31/12/2281

44. Fiona S. Atkinson, RD, Kaye Foster-Powell, RD and Jennie C. Brand-Miller, PHD. (2008, December 31). American Diabetes Association. Retrieved from International Tables of Glycemic Index and Glycemic Load Values 2008: https://care.diabetesjournals.org/content/31/12/2281

45. Editor. (2019, January 15). Diabetes.co.uk. Retrieved from Glycemic Load: www.diabetes.co.uk/diet/glycemic-load.html

46. Hite, A. (2021, February 11). Diet Doctor. Retrieved from How to Reverse Your Type 2 Diabetes: https://www.dietdoctor.com/diabetes
    Understanding the glycemic index and how to use it: https://www.wellbeing.com.au/body/health/gi-know-how.html

47. Editor. (2019, January 15). Diabetes.co.uk. Retrieved from Glycemic Load: www.diabetes.co.uk/diet/glycemic-load.html

48. Harvard TH Chan School of Public Health- The Nutrition Source. (n.d.). Retrieved from Carbohydrates and Blood Sugar: www.hsph.harvard.edu/nutritionsource/carbohydrates/carbohydrates-and-blood-sugar/

49. Harvard TH Chan School of Public Health- The Nutrition Source. (n.d.). Retrieved from Carbohydrates and Blood Sugar: www.hsph.harvard.edu/nutritionsource/carbohydrates/carbohydrates-and-blood-sugar/

50. Harvard TH Chan School of Public Health- The Nutrition Source. (n.d.). Retrieved from Carbohydrates and Blood Sugar: www.hsph.harvard.edu/nutritionsource/carbohydrates/carbohydrates-and-blood-sugar/

3. DIET PART TWO: CUTTING CARBS THE RIGHT WAY

1. What is Eatwell Everyday? | Food Standards Scotland. www.foodstandards.gov.scot/consumers/healthy-eating/eatwell/eatwell-everyday/about-eatwell-everyday/what-is-eatwell-everyday
   Hite, A. (2021, February 11). DietDoctor. Retrieved from How to Reverse Your Type 2 Diabetes: https://www.dietdoctor.com/diabetes

Food As Fuel: How to Transform Your Workout With Nutrition https://beinglike.com/food-as-fuel-how-to-transform-your-workout-with-nutrition

2. Editor. (2019, January 15). Diabetes.co.uk. Retrieved from Low Carb: https://www.diabetes.co.uk/diet/low-carb-diabetes-diet.html

3. What is Eatwell Everyday? | Food Standards Scotland. www.foodstandards.gov.scot/consumers/healthy-eating/eatwell/eatwell-everyday/about-eatwell-everyday/what-is-eatwell-everyday

Hite, A. (2021, February 11). Diet Doctor. Retrieved from How to Reverse Your Type 2 Diabetes: https://www.dietdoctor.com/diabetes

Food As Fuel: How to Transform Your Workout With Nutrition https://beinglike.com/food-as-fuel-how-to-transform-your-workout-with-nutrition

4. What is Eatwell Everyday? | Food Standards Scotland. www.foodstandards.gov.scot/consumers/healthy-eating/eatwell/eatwell-everyday/about-eatwell-everyday/what-is-eatwell-everyday

Hite, A. (2021, February 11). DietDoctor. Retrieved from How to Reverse Your Type 2 Diabetes: https://www.dietdoctor.com/diabetes

Food As Fuel: How to Transform Your Workout With Nutrition https://beinglike.com/food-as-fuel-how-to-transform-your-workout-with-nutrition/

5. What is Eatwell Everyday? | Food Standards Scotland. www.foodstandards.gov.scot/consumers/healthy-eating/eatwell/eatwell-everyday/about-eatwell-everyday/what-is-eatwell-everyday

Hite, A. (2021, February 11). DietDoctor. Retrieved from How to Reverse Your Type 2 Diabetes: https://www.dietdoctor.com/diabetes

Food As Fuel: How to Transform Your Workout With Nutrition https://beinglike.com/food-as-fuel-how-to-transform-your-workout-with-nutrition/

Kiddie, J. (2019, April 19). The Low Carb Fat Healthy Dietician. Retrieved from ADA: reducing carbs has the most evidence for improving blood sugar: https://www.lchf-rd.com/2019/04/19/

new-ada-report-reducing-carb-intake-has-most-evidence-for-improving-blood-sugar/

6. What is Eatwell Everyday? | Food Standards Scotland. www.foodstandards.gov.scot/consumers/healthy-eating/eatwell/eatwell-everyday/about-eatwell-everyday/what-is-eatwell-everyday

   Hite, A. (2021, February 11). DietDoctor. Retrieved from How to Reverse Your Type 2 Diabetes: https://www.dietdoctor.com/diabetes

   Food As Fuel: How to Transform Your Workout With Nutrition https://beinglike.com/food-as-fuel-how-to-transform-your-workout-with-nutrition/

   Kiddie, J. (2019, April 19). The Low Carb Fat Healthy Dietician. Retrieved from ADA: reducing carbs has the most evidence for improving blood sugar: https://www.lchf-rd.com/2019/04/19/new-ada-report-reducing-carb-intake-has-most-evidence-for-improving-blood-sugar/

   Snorgaard, O., Poulsen, G., Andersen, H., & A, A. (2017, February 23). PubMed.gov. Retrieved from Systematic review and meta-analysis of dietary carbohydrate restriction in patients with type 2 diabetes: https://pubmed.ncbi.nlm.nih.gov/28316796/

7. Eenfeldt, A. (2021, April 9). Diet Doctor. Retrieved from Low carb for beginners: https://www.dietdoctor.com/low-carb

   Mayo Clinic Staff. (2020, November 18). Mayo Clinic. Retrieved from Low-carb diet: Can it help you lose weight?: https://www.mayoclinic.org/healthy-lifestyle/weight-loss/in-depth/low-carb-diet/art-20045831

8. Eenfeldt, A. (2021, April 9). Diet Doctor. Retrieved from Low carb for beginners: https://www.dietdoctor.com/low-carb

9. Eenfeldt, A. (2021, April 9). Diet Doctor. Retrieved from Low carb for beginners: https://www.dietdoctor.com/low-carb

10. Eenfeldt, A. (2021, March 5). Diet Doctor. Retrieved from How low carb is low carb?: https://www.dietdoctor.com/low-carb/how-low-carb-is-low-carb

    Diabetes UK . (n.d.). Retrieved from low-carb diet and meal plan: https://www.diabetes.org.uk/guide-to-diabetes/enjoy-food/eating-with-diabetes/meal-plans/low-carb

11. Diabetes UK . (n.d.). Retrieved from low-carb diet and meal plan: https://www.diabetes.org.uk/guide-to-diabetes/enjoy-food/eating-with-diabetes/meal-plans/low-carb

12. Eenfeldt, A. (2021, April 9). Diet Doctor. Retrieved from Low carb for beginners: https://www.dietdoctor.com/low-carb

13. Eenfeldt, A. (2021, April 9). Diet Doctor. Retrieved from Low carb for beginners: https://www.dietdoctor.com/low-carb

14. Eenfeldt, A. (2021, April 9). Diet Doctor. Retrieved from Low carb for beginners: https://www.dietdoctor.com/low-carb

15. Kiddie, J. (2019, April 19). The Low Carb Fat Healthy Dietician. Retrieved from ADA: reducing carbs has the most evidence for improving blood sugar: https://www.lchf-rd.com/2019/04/19/new-ada-report-reducing-carb-intake-has-most-evidence-for-improving-blood-sugar/

16. Eenfeldt, A. (2020, December 2020). Diet Doctor. Retrieved from Low-carb fruits and berries – the best and the worst: https://www.dietdoctor.com/low-carb/fruits

17. Eenfeldt, A. (2020, December 2020). Diet Doctor. Retrieved from Low-carb fruits and berries – the best and the worst: https://www.dietdoctor.com/low-carb/fruits

18. Eenfeldt, A. (2020, December 2020). Diet Doctor. Retrieved from Low-carb fruits and berries – the best and the worst: https://www.dietdoctor.com/low-carb/fruits

19. Fletcher, J. (2020, December 22). Medical News Today. Retrieved from What can you eat on a low-carb diet?: www.medicalnewstoday.com/articles/321545

20. Fletcher, J. (2020, December 22). Medical News Today. Retrieved from What can you eat on a low-carb diet?: www.medicalnewstoday.com/articles/321545

21. Fletcher, J. (2020, December 22). Medical News Today. Retrieved from What can you eat on a low-carb diet?: www.medicalnewstoday.com/articles/321545

22. Better Homes and Gardens. (2015, June 9). Retrieved from 12 Steps to Start a Low-Carb Diet: https://www.bhg.com/recipes/healthy/eating/12-steps-to-start-a-low-carb-diet/

23. Better Homes and Gardens. (2015, June 9). Retrieved from 12 Steps to Start a Low-Carb Diet: https://www.bhg.com/recipes/healthy/eating/12-steps-to-start-a-low-carb-diet/

24. Better Homes and Gardens. (2015, June 9). Retrieved from 12 Steps to Start a Low-Carb Diet: https://www.bhg.com/recipes/healthy/eating/12-steps-to-start-a-low-carb-diet/
25. Better Homes and Gardens. (2015, June 9). Retrieved from 12 Steps to Start a Low-Carb Diet: https://www.bhg.com/recipes/healthy/eating/12-steps-to-start-a-low-carb-diet/
26. Cherrier, C. (2021, April 9). Eat Well 101. Retrieved from Baked Chicken in Foil with Asparagus and Garlic Lemon Butter Sauce: https://www.eatwell101.com/baked-chicken-in-foil-with-asparagus-recipe
27. Cherrier, C. (2021, February 9). Eat Well 101. Retrieved from Lemon Garlic Butter Steak: https://www.eatwell101.com/lemon-garlic-butter-steak-and-broccoli-skillet-recipe
28. Cherrier, C. (2021, April 10). Eat Well 101. Retrieved from Spinach Salmon Casserole with Cream Cheese and Mozzarella: https://www.eatwell101.com/spinach-salmon-casserole-recipe
29. Cherrier, C. (2021, February 24). Eat Well 101. Retrieved from Instant Pot Keto Tuscan Soup: https://www.eatwell101.com/instant-pot-keto-tuscan-soup-recipe
30. Cherrier, C. (2020, November 3). Eat Well 101. Retrieved from Creamy Broccoli and Cauliflower Stir-Fry with Sun-dried Tomatoes: https://www.eatwell101.com/creamy-broccoli-cauliflower-recipe
31. Cherrier, C. (2020, October 8). Eat Well 101. Retrieved from Healthy Tomato Zucchini Soup {Vegan + Gluten-Free}: https://www.eatwell101.com/tomato-zucchini-soup-recipe
32. Cherrier, C. (2020, August 2). Eat Well 101. Retrieved from Honey Balsamic Pan-Seared Cabbage Steaks: https://www.eatwell101.com/honey-balsamic-cabbage-steaks-recipe
33. Cherrier, C. (2020, August 7). Eat Well 101. Retrieved from Lemon Garlic Butter Zucchini Noodles: https://www.eatwell101.com/garlic-butter-zucchini-noodles-recipe
34. Cherrier, C. (2021, March 4). Eat Well 101. Retrieved from Brown Butter Garlic Cauliflower Foil Packets: https://www.eatwell101.com/cauliflower-foil-packets-recipe

4. FASTING IS YOUR FRIEND: A QUICK GUIDE TO INTERMITTENT FASTING

1. Albosta, M., & Bakke, C. (2021, February 3). Clinical Diabetes and Endocrinology. Retrieved from Intermittent fasting: is there a role in the treatment of diabetes? A review of the literature and guide for primary care physicians: https://clindiabetesendo.biomedcentral.com/articles/10.1186/s40842-020-00116-1

2. Albosta, M., & Bakke, C. (2021, February 3). Clinical Diabetes and Endocrinology. Retrieved from Intermittent fasting: is there a role in the treatment of diabetes? A review of the literature and guide for primary care physicians: https://clindiabetesendo.biomedcentral.com/articles/10.1186/s40842-020-00116-1

3. Furmli, S., Elmasry, R., Ramos, M., & Fung, J. (2017). BMJ Case Reports. Retrieved from Therapeutic use of intermittent fasting for people with type 2 diabetes as an alternative to insulin: https://casereports.bmj.com/content/2018/bcr-2017-221854

    8 Tricks To Get Rid of Stubborn Love Handle: https://www.thealternativedaily.com/8-tricks-to-get-rid-of-stubborn-love-handles/

    Shomon, M. (2019, October 28). Health Central. Retrieved from Will Intermittent Fasting Help Your Type 2 Diabetes?: https://www.healthcentral.com/slideshow/will-intermittent-fasting-help-your-type-2-diabetes

4. Albosta, M., & Bakke, C. (2021, February 3). Clinical Diabetes and Endocrinology. Retrieved from Intermittent fasting: is there a role in the treatment of diabetes? A review of the literature and guide for primary care physicians: https://clindiabetesendo.biomedcentral.com/articles/10.1186/s40842-020-00116-1

5. Shomon, M. (2019, October 28). Health Central. Retrieved from Will Intermittent Fasting Help Your Type 2 Diabetes?: https://www.healthcentral.com/slideshow/will-intermittent-fasting-help-your-type-2-diabetes

6. Shomon, M. (2019, October 28). Health Central. Retrieved from Will Intermittent Fasting Help Your Type 2 Diabetes?: https://www.healthcentral.com/slideshow/will-intermittent-fasting-help-your-type-2-diabetes

7. Shomon, M. (2019, October 28). Health Central. Retrieved from Will Intermittent Fasting Help Your Type 2 Diabetes?: https://www.healthcentral.com/slideshow/will-intermittent-fasting-help-your-type-2-diabetes

8. Shomon, M. (2019, October 28). Health Central. Retrieved from Will Intermittent Fasting Help Your Type 2 Diabetes?: https://www.healthcentral.com/slideshow/will-intermittent-fasting-help-your-type-2-diabetes

9. Furmli, S., Elmasry, R., Ramos, M., & Fung, J. (2017). BMJ Case Reports. Retrieved from Therapeutic use of intermittent fasting for people with type 2 diabetes as an alternative to insulin: https://casereports.bmj.com/content/2018/bcr-2017-221854
8 Tricks To Get Rid of Stubborn Love Handle: https://www.thealternativedaily.com/8-tricks-to-get-rid-of-stubborn-love-handles/

10. Furmli, S., Elmasry, R., Ramos, M., & Fung, J. (2017). BMJ Case Reports. Retrieved from Therapeutic use of intermittent fasting for people with type 2 diabetes as an alternative to insulin: https://casereports.bmj.com/content/2018/bcr-2017-221854
8 Tricks To Get Rid of Stubborn Love Handle: https://www.thealternativedaily.com/8-tricks-to-get-rid-of-stubborn-love-handles/

11. Shomon, M. (2019, October 28). Health Central. Retrieved from Will Intermittent Fasting Help Your Type 2 Diabetes?: https://www.healthcentral.com/slideshow/will-intermittent-fasting-help-your-type-2-diabetes
Tello, M. (2018, June 29). Harvard Health Publishing. Retrieved from Intermittent fasting: Surprising update: www.health.harvard.edu/blog/intermittent-fasting-surprising-update-2018062914156

12. Tello, M. (2018, June 29). Harvard Health Publishing. Retrieved from Intermittent fasting: Surprising update: www.health.harvard.edu/blog/intermittent-fasting-surprising-update-2018062914156

13. Editor. (2019, January 15). Diabetes.co.uk. Retrieved from 5:2 Fasting Diet: https://www.diabetes.co.uk/diet/5-2-intermittent-fast-diet.html

14. Johnson, J. (2018, January 28). Medical News Today. Retrieved from How to do the 5:2 diet: https://www.medicalnewstoday.com/articles/324303

15. Johnson, J. (2018, January 28). Medical News Today. Retrieved from How to do the 5:2 diet: https://www.medicalnewstoday.com/articles/324303

16. Silver, N. (2019, March 29). Healthline. Retrieved from What Happens If You Don't Eat for a Day?: https://www.healthline.com/health/food-nutrition/what-happens-if-you-dont-eat-for-a-day
   Post Workout: How to Take Care of Your Body - Living Smart: https://livingsmartgirl.com/post-workout-how-to-take-care-of-your-body/

17. Silver, N. (2019, March 29). Healthline. Retrieved from What Happens If You Don't Eat for a Day?: https://www.healthline.com/health/food-nutrition/what-happens-if-you-dont-eat-for-a-day
   Post Workout: How to Take Care of Your Body - Living Smart: https://livingsmartgirl.com/post-workout-how-to-take-care-of-your-body/

18. Silver, N. (2019, March 29). Healthline. Retrieved from What Happens If You Don't Eat for a Day?: https://www.healthline.com/health/food-nutrition/what-happens-if-you-dont-eat-for-a-day
   Post Workout: How to Take Care of Your Body - Living Smart: https://livingsmartgirl.com/post-workout-how-to-take-care-of-your-body/

19. Silver, N. (2019, March 29). Healthline. Retrieved from What Happens If You Don't Eat for a Day?: https://www.healthline.com/health/food-nutrition/what-happens-if-you-dont-eat-for-a-day
   Post Workout: How to Take Care of Your Body - Living Smart: https://livingsmartgirl.com/post-workout-how-to-take-care-of-your-body/

20. Mommers, H. (2020, October 26). Our Green Health. Retrieved from The Benefits of Water for the Human Body. Source of Life: https://ourgreenhealth.com/water-for-the-human-body/#

21. Silver, N. (2019, March 29). Healthline. Retrieved from What Happens If You Don't Eat for a Day?: https://www.healthline.com/health/food-nutrition/what-happens-if-you-dont-eat-for-a-day

Post Workout: How to Take Care of Your Body - Living Smart: https://livingsmartgirl.com/post-workout-how-to-take-care-of-your-body/

22. Kubala, J. (2020, July 1). Healthline. Retrieved from Is Eating One Meal a Day a Safe and Effective Way to Lose Weight?: www. healthline.com/health/one-meal-a-day

23. Kubala, J. (2020, July 1). Healthline. Retrieved from Is Eating One Meal a Day a Safe and Effective Way to Lose Weight?: www. healthline.com/health/one-meal-a-day

24. Kubala, J. (2020, July 1). Healthline. Retrieved from Is Eating One Meal a Day a Safe and Effective Way to Lose Weight?: www. healthline.com/health/one-meal-a-day

25. Shomon, M. (2019, October 28). Health Central. Retrieved from Will Intermittent Fasting Help Your Type 2 Diabetes?: https://www. healthcentral.com/slideshow/will-intermittent-fasting-help-your-type-2-diabetes

26. Tinsley, G. (2017, September 17). Healthline. Retrieved from Time-Restricted Eating: A Beginner's Guide: https://www.healthline. com/nutrition/time-restricted-eating

27. Tinsley, G. (2017, September 17). Healthline. Retrieved from Time-Restricted Eating: A Beginner's Guide: https://www.healthline. com/nutrition/time-restricted-eating

28. Tinsley, G. (2017, September 17). Healthline. Retrieved from Time-Restricted Eating: A Beginner's Guide: https://www.healthline. com/nutrition/time-restricted-eating

5. LOSING WEIGHT (YOU'RE ALREADY ON YOUR WAY!)

1. Doheny, K. (2018, October 26). Endocrineweb. Retrieved from Reversing Diabetes with Weight Loss: Stronger Evidence, Bigger Payoff: www.endocrineweb.com/news/diabetes/60067-reversing-diabetes-weight-loss-stronger-evidence-bigger-payoff

Ryan, E., & McDermott, J. (2019, March 22). diaTribeLearn. Retrieved from Type 2 Diabetes Remission: What is it and How Can it be Done?: https://diatribe.org/type-2-diabetes-remission-what-it-and-how-can-it-be-done

2. Doheny, K. (2018, October 26). Endocrineweb. Retrieved from Reversing Diabetes with Weight Loss: Stronger Evidence, Bigger Payoff: www.endocrineweb.com/news/diabetes/60067-reversing-diabetes-weight-loss-stronger-evidence-bigger-payoff

Ryan, E., & McDermott, J. (2019, March 22). diaTribeLearn. Retrieved from Type 2 Diabetes Remission: What is it and How Can it be Done?: https://diatribe.org/type-2-diabetes-remission-what-it-and-how-can-it-be-done

Lena, M., Leslie, W., Barnes, A., Brosnahan, N., Thom, G., L, M., et al. (2017). Primary care-led weight management for remission of type 2 diabetes (DiRECT): an open-label, cluster- randomized trial. The Lancet, 541-551. Retrieved from https://www.thelancet.com/journals/lancet/article/PIIS0140-6736(17)33102-1/fulltext

3. Doheny, K. (2018, October 26). Endocrineweb. Retrieved from Reversing Diabetes with Weight Loss: Stronger Evidence, Bigger Payoff: www.endocrineweb.com/news/diabetes/60067-reversing-diabetes-weight-loss-stronger-evidence-bigger-payoff

Ryan, E., & McDermott, J. (2019, March 22). diaTribeLearn. Retrieved from Type 2 Diabetes Remission: What is it and How Can it be Done?: https://diatribe.org/type-2-diabetes-remission-what-it-and-how-can-it-be-done

Lena, M., Leslie, W., Barnes, A., Brosnahan, N., Thom, G., L, M., et al. (2017). Primary care-led weight management for remission of type 2 diabetes (DiRECT): an open-label, cluster- randomized trial. The Lancet, 541-551. Retrieved from https://www.thelancet.com/journals/lancet/article/PIIS0140-6736(17)33102-1/fulltext

4. Doheny, K. (2018, October 26). Endocrineweb. Retrieved from Reversing Diabetes with Weight Loss: Stronger Evidence, Bigger Payoff: www.endocrineweb.com/news/diabetes/60067-reversing-diabetes-weight-loss-stronger-evidence-bigger-payoff

5. Doheny, K. (2018, October 26). Endocrineweb. Retrieved from Reversing Diabetes with Weight Loss: Stronger Evidence, Bigger Payoff: www.endocrineweb.com/news/diabetes/60067-reversing-diabetes-weight-loss-stronger-evidence-bigger-payoff

6. Doheny, K. (2018, October 26). Endocrineweb. Retrieved from Reversing Diabetes with Weight Loss: Stronger Evidence, Bigger Payoff: www.endocrineweb.com/news/diabetes/60067-reversing-diabetes-weight-loss-stronger-evidence-bigger-payoff

MacMillan, A. (n.d.). Time. Retrieved from How Weight Loss Can Reverse Type 2 Diabetes: https://time.com/collection/guide-to-weight-loss/4940354/reverse-diabetes-weight-loss/

7. Doheny, K. (2018, October 26). Endocrineweb. Retrieved from Reversing Diabetes with Weight Loss: Stronger Evidence, Bigger Payoff: www.endocrineweb.com/news/diabetes/60067-reversing-diabetes-weight-loss-stronger-evidence-bigger-payoff

MacMillan, A. (n.d.). Time. Retrieved from How Weight Loss Can Reverse Type 2 Diabetes: https://time.com/collection/guide-to-weight-loss/4940354/reverse-diabetes-weight-loss/

8. Johns Hopkins Medicine. (2013, July 16). Retrieved from People With Pre-Diabetes Who Drop Substantial Weight May Ward Off Type 2 Diabetes: www.hopkinsmedicine.org/news/media/releases/people_with_pre_diabetes_who_drop_substantial_weight_may_ward_off_type_2_diabetes

9. Krans, B. (2020, June 29). Healthline. Retrieved from Balanced Diet: https://www.healthline.com/health/balanced-diet#what-to-eat

10. Harvard TH Chan School of Public Health- The Nutrition Source. (n.d.). Retrieved from Carbohydrates and Blood Sugar: https://www.hsph.harvard.edu/nutritionsource/carbohydrates/carbohydrates-and-blood-sugar/

Fiona S. Atkinson, RD, Kaye Foster-Powell, RD and Jennie C. Brand-Miller, PHD. (2008, December 31). American Diabetes Association. Retrieved from International Tables of Glycemic Index and Glycemic Load Values 2008: https://care.diabetesjournals.org/content/31/12/2281

11. Eenfeldt, A. (2021, April 9). Diet Doctor. Retrieved from Low carb for beginners: https://www.dietdoctor.com/low-carb

Diabetes UK . (n.d.). Retrieved from low-carb diet and meal plan: https://www.diabetes.org.uk/guide-to-diabetes/enjoy-food/eating-with-diabetes/meal-plans/low-carb

12. Shomon, M. (2019, October 28). Health Central. Retrieved from Will Intermittent Fasting Help Your Type 2 Diabetes?: www.healthcentral.com/slideshow/will-intermittent-fasting-help-your-type-2-diabetes

Tello, M. (2018, June 29). Harvard Health Publishing. Retrieved from Intermittent fasting: Surprising update: www.health.harvard.edu/blog/intermittent-fasting-surprising-update-2018062914156

13. Tello, M. (2018, June 29). Harvard Health Publishing. Retrieved from Intermittent fasting: Surprising update: www.health.harvard.edu/blog/intermittent-fasting-surprising-update-2018062914156

14. Raman, R. (2019, August 5). Healthline. Retrieved from The 8 Best Diet Plans — Sustainability, Weight Loss, and More: www.healthline.com/nutrition/best-diet-plans#TOC_TITLE_HDR_5

15. Staff, M. C. (2020, August 25). Mayo Clinic- Healthy lifestyle. Retrieved from Paleo diet: What is it and why is it so popular?: www.mayoclinic.org/healthy-lifestyle/nutrition-and-healthy-eating/in-depth/paleo-diet/art-20111182

16. Raman, R. (2019, August 5). Healthline. Retrieved from The 8 Best Diet Plans — Sustainability, Weight Loss, and More: www.healthline.com/nutrition/best-diet-plans#TOC_TITLE_HDR_5

    Editor. (2019, January 15). Diabetes.co.uk- Nutrition. Retrieved from Fats and Diabetes: www.diabetes.co.uk/nutrition/fat-and-diabetes.html

17. Raman, R. (2019, August 5). Healthline. Retrieved from The 8 Best Diet Plans — Sustainability, Weight Loss, and More: www.healthline.com/nutrition/best-diet-plans#TOC_TITLE_HDR_5

    Carroll, C. (2021, March 25). VeryWellFit. Retrieved from Pros and Cons of the Mediterranean Diet: www.verywellfit.com/the-mediterranean-diet-pros-and-cons-4685664

18. Raman, R. (2019, August 5). Healthline. Retrieved from The 8 Best Diet Plans — Sustainability, Weight Loss, and More: www.healthline.com/nutrition/best-diet-plans#TOC_TITLE_HDR_5

    Kubala, J. (2018, March 13). Healthline. Retrieved from Weight Watchers Diet Review: Does It Work for Weight Loss?: https://www.healthline.com/nutrition/weight-watchers-diet-review

19. Raman, R. (2019, August 5). Healthline. Retrieved from The 8 Best Diet Plans — Sustainability, Weight Loss, and More: www.healthline.com/nutrition/best-diet-plans#TOC_TITLE_HDR_5

    Editor. (2019, January 15). Diabetes.co.uk. Retrieved from DASH Diet – Dietary Approaches to Stop Hypertension Diet: www.diabetes.co.uk/diet/dash-diet.html

6. THE POWER OF REGULAR EXERCISE
(AND HOW YOU CAN MAKE IT A HABIT)

1. Cooper Aerobics. (n.d.). Retrieved from Kenneth H. Cooper, MD, MPH Full Bio: https://cooperaerobics.com/About/Our-Leaders/Kenneth-H-Cooper,-MD,-MPH.aspx
2. Harvard Health Publishing. (2021, February 2021). Retrieved from The importance of exercise when you have diabetes: www.health.harvard.edu/staying-healthy/the-importance-of-exercise-when-you-have-diabetes
3. Taylor, R., Al-Mrabeh, A., & Sattar, N. (2019, September 7). PubMed.gov. Retrieved from Understanding the mechanisms of reversal of type 2 diabetes: https://pubmed.ncbi.nlm.nih.gov/31097391
4. Diabetes Care Community. (n.d.). Retrieved from Can exercise cure or reverse diabetes?: www.diabetescarecommunity.ca/diet-and-fitness-articles/physical-activity-articles/can-exercise-cure-or-reverse-diabetes/
5. Raman, R. (2017, May 17). Healthline. Retrieved from 14 Natural Ways to Improve Your Insulin Sensitivity: www.healthline.com/nutrition/improve-insulin-sensitivity#TOC_TITLE_HDR_4
6. Encyclopedia of Children's Health. (n.d.). Retrieved from Exercise: www.healthofchildren.com/E-F/Exercise.html
7. Colberg, S; Sigal, R.J; Yardley, J.E et al. (2016, November). Diabetes Care. Retrieved from Physical Activity/Exercise and Diabetes: A Position Statement of the American Diabetes Association: https://care.diabetesjournals.org/content/39/11/2065 Frontiers I Glycemic and Metabolic Effects of Two Long: www.frontiersin.org/articles/10.3389/fendo.2017.00154/full
8. Colberg, S; Sigal, R.J; Yardley, J.E et al. (2016, November). Diabetes Care. Retrieved from Physical Activity/Exercise and Diabetes: A Position Statement of the American Diabetes Association: https://care.diabetesjournals.org/content/39/11/2065 Frontiers I Glycemic and Metabolic Effects of Two Long: www.frontiersin.org/articles/10.3389/fendo.2017.00154/full
9. Weil, R. (2021, January 7). MedicineNet. Retrieved from Aerobic Exercise: Types, List, and Benefits: https://www.medicinenet.com/aerobic_exercise/article.htm

10. Colberg, S; Sigal, R.J; Yardley, J.E et al. (2016, November). Diabetes Care. Retrieved from Physical Activity/Exercise and Diabetes: A Position Statement of the American Diabetes Association:, https://care.diabetesjournals.org/content/39/11/2065 Frontiers | Glycemic and Metabolic Effects of Two Long: www.frontiersin.org/articles/10.3389/fendo.2017.00154/full

11. Colberg, S; Sigal, R.J; Yardley, J.E et al. (2016, November). Diabetes Care. Retrieved from Physical Activity/Exercise and Diabetes: A Position Statement of the American Diabetes Association: https://care.diabetesjournals.org/content/39/11/2065 Frontiers | Glycemic and Metabolic Effects of Two Long: www.frontiersin.org/articles/10.3389/fendo.2017.00154/full

12. Ricketts, D. (2020, August 21). Study.com. Retrieved from Anaerobic Exercise: Definition, Benefits & Examples: https://study.com/academy/lesson/anaerobic-exercise-definition-benefits-examples.html

13. Colberg, S; Sigal, R.J; Yardley, J.E et al. (2016, November). Diabetes Care. Retrieved from Physical Activity/Exercise and Diabetes: A Position Statement of the American Diabetes Association: https://care.diabetesjournals.org/content/39/11/2065 Frontiers | Glycemic and Metabolic Effects of Two Long: www.frontiersin.org/articles/10.3389/fendo.2017.00154/full

14. Colberg, S; Sigal, R.J; Yardley, J.E et al. (2016, November). Diabetes Care. Retrieved from Physical Activity/Exercise and Diabetes: A Position Statement of the American Diabetes Association: https://care.diabetesjournals.org/content/39/11/2065 Frontiers | Glycemic and Metabolic Effects of Two Long: www.frontiersin.org/articles/10.3389/fendo.2017.00154/full

15. Colberg, S; Sigal, R.J; Yardley, J.E et al. (2016, November). Diabetes Care. Retrieved from Physical Activity/Exercise and Diabetes: A Position Statement of the American Diabetes Association: https://care.diabetesjournals.org/content/39/11/2065 Frontiers | Glycemic and Metabolic Effects of Two Long: www.frontiersin.org/articles/10.3389/fendo.2017.00154/full

16. Colberg, S; Sigal, R.J; Yardley, J.E et al. (2016, November). Diabetes Care. Retrieved from Physical Activity/Exercise and Diabetes: A Position Statement of the American Diabetes Association: https://care.diabetesjournals.org/content/39/11/2065

Frontiers | Glycemic and Metabolic Effects of Two Long: www.
frontiersin.org/articles/10.3389/fendo.2017.00154/full

17. Colberg, S; Sigal, R.J; Yardley, J.E et al. (2016, November). Diabetes
Care. Retrieved from Physical Activity/Exercise and Diabetes: A
Position Statement of the American Diabetes Association:
https://care.diabetesjournals.org/content/39/11/2065
Frontiers | Glycemic and Metabolic Effects of Two Long: www.
frontiersin.org/articles/10.3389/fendo.2017.00154/full

18. Colberg, S; Sigal, R.J; Yardley, J.E et al. (2016, November). Diabetes
Care. Retrieved from Physical Activity/Exercise and Diabetes: A
Position Statement of the American Diabetes Association:
https://care.diabetesjournals.org/content/39/11/2065
Frontiers | Glycemic and Metabolic Effects of Two Long: www.
frontiersin.org/articles/10.3389/fendo.2017.00154/full

19. Editor. (2018, July 31). Diabetes.co.uk. Retrieved from Importance
of exercise emphasized in new prediabetes study: www.diabetes.co.
uk/news/2018/jul/importance-of-exercise-emphasised-in-new-
prediabetes-study-98501208.html

20. MacDonald, CS; Johansen, MY; Nielsen SM; et al. (2020, March).
PubMed.gov. Retrieved from Dose-Response Effects of Exercise on
Glucose-Lowering Medications for Type 2 Diabetes: A Secondary
Analysis of a Randomized Clinical Trial: https://pubmed.ncbi.nlm.
nih.gov/32007295/

21. Fetters, KA. (2020, September 15). Everyday Health. Retrieved from
How Exercise Helps Prevent and Manage Type 2 Diabetes: www.
everydayhealth.com/type-2-diabetes/how-exercise-helps-prevent-
and-manage-type-2-diabetes/

22. Fetters, KA. (2020, September 15). Everyday Health. Retrieved from
How Exercise Helps Prevent and Manage Type 2 Diabetes: www.
everydayhealth.com/type-2-diabetes/how-exercise-helps-prevent-
and-manage-type-2-diabetes/

23. Fetters, KA. (2020, September 15). Everyday Health. Retrieved from
How Exercise Helps Prevent and Manage Type 2 Diabetes: www.
everydayhealth.com/type-2-diabetes/how-exercise-helps-prevent-
and-manage-type-2-diabetes/

24. Fetters, KA. (2020, September 15). Everyday Health. Retrieved from
How Exercise Helps Prevent and Manage Type 2 Diabetes: www.
everydayhealth.com/type-2-diabetes/how-exercise-helps-prevent-
and-manage-type-2-diabetes/

25. Fetters, KA. (2020, September 15). Everyday Health. Retrieved from How Exercise Helps Prevent and Manage Type 2 Diabetes: www. everydayhealth.com/type-2-diabetes/how-exercise-helps-prevent-and-manage-type-2-diabetes/

26. Cathe. (n.d.). Retrieved from What Role Does Exercise Play in Reversing Pre-diabetes?: https://cathe.com/what-role-does-exercise-play-in-reversing-pre-diabetes/

27. Cathe. (n.d.). Retrieved from What Role Does Exercise Play in Reversing Pre-diabetes?: https://cathe.com/what-role-does-exercise-play-in-reversing-pre-diabetes/

28. Cathe. (n.d.). Retrieved from What Role Does Exercise Play in Reversing Pre-diabetes?:

    https://cathe.com/what-role-does-exercise-play-in-reversing-pre-diabetes/

    Colberg, S; Sigal, R.J; Yardley, J.E et al. (2016, November). Diabetes Care. Retrieved from Physical Activity/Exercise and Diabetes: A Position Statement of the American Diabetes Association:

    https://care.diabetesjournals.org/content/39/11/2065

    Frontiers | Glycemic and Metabolic Effects of Two Long: www. frontiersin.org/articles/10.3389/fendo.2017.00154/full

29. Cathe. (n.d.). Retrieved from What Role Does Exercise Play in Reversing Pre-diabetes?:

    https://cathe.com/what-role-does-exercise-play-in-reversing-pre-diabetes/

    Colberg, S; Sigal, R.J; Yardley, J.E et al. (2016, November). Diabetes Care. Retrieved from Physical Activity/Exercise and Diabetes: A Position Statement of the American Diabetes Association:

    https://care.diabetesjournals.org/content/39/11/2065

    Frontiers | Glycemic and Metabolic Effects of Two Long: www. frontiersin.org/articles/10.3389/fendo.2017.00154/full

30. Fetters, KA. (2020, September 15). Everyday Health. Retrieved from How Exercise Helps Prevent and Manage Type 2 Diabetes: www. everydayhealth.com/type-2-diabetes/how-exercise-helps-prevent-and-manage-type-2-diabetes/

31. Hanley, T. (2019, April 17). Tiege. Retrieved from How Long Does It Take to Create a Habit?: https://www.tiege.com/blogs/news/how-long-does-it-take-to-create-a-habit

RESOURCES | 219

32. Mackay, B; Mackay, K. (2021, April 5). The Art of Manliness. Retrieved from The 10 Best Ways to Make Exercise an Unbreakable Habit: www.artofmanliness.com/articles/10-best-tactics-making-exercise-unbreakable-habit/

33. Mackay, B; Mackay, K. (2021, April 5). The Art of Manliness. Retrieved from The 10 Best Ways to Make Exercise an Unbreakable Habit: www.artofmanliness.com/articles/10-best-tactics-making-exercise-unbreakable-habit/

34. Mackay, B; Mackay, K. (2021, April 5). The Art of Manliness. Retrieved from The 10 Best Ways to Make Exercise an Unbreakable Habit: www.artofmanliness.com/articles/10-best-tactics-making-exercise-unbreakable-habit/

35. Mackay, B; Mackay, K. (2021, April 5). The Art of Manliness. Retrieved from The 10 Best Ways to Make Exercise an Unbreakable Habit: www.artofmanliness.com/articles/10-best-tactics-making-exercise-unbreakable-habit/

36. Mackay, B; Mackay, K. (2021, April 5). The Art of Manliness. Retrieved from The 10 Best Ways to Make Exercise an Unbreakable Habit: www.artofmanliness.com/articles/10-best-tactics-making-exercise-unbreakable-habit/

37. Mackay, B; Mackay, K. (2021, April 5). The Art of Manliness. Retrieved from The 10 Best Ways to Make Exercise an Unbreakable Habit: www.artofmanliness.com/articles/10-best-tactics-making-exercise-unbreakable-habit/

38. Mackay, B; Mackay, K. (2021, April 5). The Art of Manliness. Retrieved from The 10 Best Ways to Make Exercise an Unbreakable Habit: www.artofmanliness.com/articles/10-best-tactics-making-exercise-unbreakable-habit/

39. Mackay, B; Mackay, K. (2021, April 5). The Art of Manliness. Retrieved from The 10 Best Ways to Make Exercise an Unbreakable Habit: www.artofmanliness.com/articles/10-best-tactics-making-exercise-unbreakable-habit/

7. THE SECRETS OF HYDRATION-AND HOW TO DO IT RIGHT

1. Popkin, B., & D'Anci K, R. I. (2010, August 1). Water, Hydration and Health. Nutrition Reviews, 439-458. Retrieved from https:// academic.oup.com/nutritionreviews/article/68/8/439/1841926

2. Stavros, K., & Costas, A. (2010, November). Water Physiology. Nutrition Today, 27-32. https://doi.org/10.1097/NT.0b013e3181fe1713

3. Popkin, B., & D'Anci K, R. I. (2010, August 1). Water, Hydration and Health. Nutrition Reviews, 439-458. Retrieved from https:// academic.oup.com/nutritionreviews/article/68/8/439/1841926

4. Stavros, K., & Costas, A. (2010, November). Water Physiology. Nutrition Today, 27-32. https://doi.org/10.1097/NT.0b013e3181fe1713

5. Stavros, K., & Costas, A. (2010, November). Water Physiology. Nutrition Today, 27-32. https://doi.org/10.1097/NT.0b013e3181fe1713

6. Stavros, K., & Costas, A. (2010, November). Water Physiology. Nutrition Today, 27-32. https://doi.org/10.1097/NT.0b013e3181fe1713

7. Stavros, K., & Costas, A. (2010, November). Water Physiology. Nutrition Today, 27-32. https://doi.org/10.1097/NT.0b013e3181fe1713

8. Stavros, K., & Costas, A. (2010, November). Water Physiology. Nutrition Today, 27-32. https://doi.org/10.1097/NT.0b013e3181fe1713

9. Popkin, B., & D'Anci K, R. I. (2010, August 1). Water, Hydration and Health. Nutrition Reviews, 439-458. Retrieved from https:// academic.oup.com/nutritionreviews/article/68/8/439/1841926

10. Popkin, B., & D'Anci K, R. I. (2010, August 1). Water, Hydration and Health. Nutrition Reviews, 439-458. Retrieved from https:// academic.oup.com/nutritionreviews/article/68/8/439/1841926
    Steven, E. (2020, June 9). Livestrong.com. Retrieved from What Really Happens to Your Body When You're Dehydrated: www. livestrong.com/article/13726071-dehydration-effects/

11. Popkin, B., & D'Anci K, R. I. (2010, August 1). Water, Hydration and Health. Nutrition Reviews, 439-458. Retrieved from https://academic.oup.com/nutritionreviews/article/68/8/439/1841926
   Steven, E. (2020, June 9). Livestrong.com. Retrieved from What Really Happens to Your Body When You're Dehydrated: www.livestrong.com/article/13726071-dehydration-effects/

12. Steven, E. (2020, June 9). Livestrong.com. Retrieved from What Really Happens to Your Body When You're Dehydrated: www.livestrong.com/article/13726071-dehydration-effects/

13. Popkin, B., & D'Anci K, R. I. (2010, August 1). Water, Hydration and Health. Nutrition Reviews, 439-458. Retrieved from https://academic.oup.com/nutritionreviews/article/68/8/439/1841926

14. Editor. (2019, January 15). Diabetes.co.uk. Retrieved from Dehydration and Diabetes: www.diabetes.co.uk/dehydration-and-diabetes.html

15. Popkin, B., & D'Anci K, R. I. (2010, August 1). Water, Hydration and Health. Nutrition Reviews, 439-458. Retrieved from https://academic.oup.com/nutritionreviews/article/68/8/439/1841926

16. Roussel, R., Fezeu, L., Bouby, N; et al. (2011, December). American Diabetes Association. Retrieved from Low Water Intake and Risk for New-Onset Hyperglycaemia: https://care.diabetesjournals.org/content/34/12/2551.full

17. Oerum, C. (2019, May 15). Diabetesrong. Retrieved from Water and Diabetes: Are You Drinking Enough Water?: https://diabetesstrong.com/water-diabetes-drinking-enough-water/

18. Spira, A., Gowrishankar, M., Halperin, M; et al. (1997, December). Factors contributing to the degree of polyuria in a patient with poorly controlled diabetes mellitus. AJKD, 829- 835. Retrieved from https://www.ajkd.org/article/S0272-6386(97)90089-5/pdf

19. Oerum, C. (2019, May 15). Diabetesrong. Retrieved from Water and Diabetes: Are You Drinking Enough Water?: https://diabetesstrong.com/water-diabetes-drinking-enough-water/

20. Oerum, C. (2019, May 15). Diabetesrong. Retrieved from Water and Diabetes: Are You Drinking Enough Water?: https://diabetesstrong.com/water-diabetes-drinking-enough-water/

21. Oerum, C. (2019, May 15). Diabetesrong. Retrieved from Water and Diabetes: Are You Drinking Enough Water?: https://diabetesstrong.com/water-diabetes-drinking-enough-water/

22. Vieira, G. (2020, January 7). Insulin In Nation. Retrieved from How Drinking Plenty of Water Improves Your Diabetes Health: https://

insulinnation.com/living/how-drinking-plenty-of-water-improves-your-diabetes-health/

Pietrangelo, A. (2018, September 28). Healthline. Retrieved from The Effects of Caffeine on Your Body: https://www.healthline.com/health/caffeine-effects-on-body#Central-nervous-system

23. Vieira, G. (2020, January 7). Insulin In Nation. Retrieved from How Drinking Plenty of Water Improves Your Diabetes Health: https://insulinnation.com/living/how-drinking-plenty-of-water-improves-your-diabetes-health/

10.Hugues, S. (2021, February 5). Very Well Health. Retrieved from The Best Beverages for People with Diabetes: https://www.verywellhealth.com/what-to-drink-when-you-have-diabetes-1087162

24. Santos- Longhurst, A. (2019, March 8). Healthline. Retrieved from Diabetes, Alcohol, and Social Drinking: www.healthline.com/health/type-2-diabetes/facts-diabetes-alcohol#5.-Alcohol-can-cause-hypoglycemia

25. American Diabetes Association. (n.d.). Retrieved from Alcohol & Diabetes: www.diabetes.org/healthy-living/medication-treatments/alcohol-diabetes

26. https://www.cancerresearchuk.org/about-cancer/causes-of-cancer/alcohol-and-cancer/does-alcohol-cause-cancer

27. https://www.cancerresearchuk.org/about-cancer/causes-of-cancer/alcohol-and-cancer/does-alcohol-cause-cancer

28. https://www.cancerresearchuk.org/about-cancer/causes-of-cancer/alcohol-and-cancer/does-alcohol-cause-cancer

29. https://www.cancerresearchuk.org/about-cancer/causes-of-cancer/alcohol-and-cancer/does-alcohol-cause-cancer

30. American Addiction Centers. (2021, March 30). Retrieved from Alcohol & Diabetes: Can Alcohol Cause Diabetes?: https://americanaddictioncenters.org/alcoholism-treatment/alcohol-abuse-and-diabetes

31. Diabetes UK. (n.d.). Retrieved from Alcohol and Diabetes: www.diabetes.org.uk/guide-to-diabetes/enjoy-food/what-to-drink-with-diabetes/alcohol-and-diabetes

Elliott, S. (2017, July 27). Healthfully. Retrieved from How Much Water Should a Type 2 Diabetic Drink?: https://healthfully.com/much-should-type-diabetic-drink-5316990.html

32. Vieira, G. (2020, January 7). Insulin In Nation. Retrieved from How Drinking Plenty of Water Improves Your Diabetes Health: https://insulinnation.com/living/how-drinking-plenty-of-water-improves-your-diabetes-health/

33. Diabetes UK. (n.d.). Retrieved from Alcohol and Diabetes: www.diabetes.org.uk/guide-to-diabetes/enjoy-food/what-to-drink-with-diabetes/alcohol-and-diabetes
Elliott, S. (2017, July 27). Healthfully. Retrieved from How Much Water Should a Type 2 Diabetic Drink?: https://healthfully.com/much-should-type-diabetic-drink-5316990.html

8. SLEEP: THE FORGOTTEN COMPONENT OF GOOD HEALTH

1. Brinkman, J., Reddy, V., & Sharma, S. (2021, April 19). PubMed.gov. Retrieved from Physiology of Sleep: https://pubmed.ncbi.nlm.nih.gov/29494118/

2. Physiopedia. (n.d.). Retrieved from Sleep: Theory, Function, and Physiology:
https://www.physio-pedia.com/Sleep:_Theory,_Function_and_Physiology#cite_ref-:3_2-0

3. Physiopedia. (n.d.). Retrieved from Sleep: Theory, Function, and Physiology:
https://www.physio-pedia.com/Sleep:_Theory,_Function_and_Physiology#cite_ref-:3_2-0

4. Suni, E. (2020, September 25). Sleep Foundation. Retrieved from Circadian Rhythm: https://www.sleepfoundation.org/circadian-rhythm

5. NIH. (n.d.). Retrieved from Brain Basics: Understanding Sleep: www.ninds.nih.gov/Disorders/Patient-Caregiver-Education/Understanding-Sleep

6. NIH. (n.d.). Retrieved from Brain Basics: Understanding Sleep: www.ninds.nih.gov/Disorders/Patient-Caregiver-Education/Understanding-Sleep

7. NIH. (n.d.). Retrieved from Brain Basics: Understanding Sleep: www.ninds.nih.gov/Disorders/Patient-Caregiver-Education/Understanding-Sleep

8. NIH. (n.d.). Retrieved from Brain Basics: Understanding Sleep: www.ninds.nih.gov/Disorders/Patient-Caregiver-Education/ Understanding-Sleep

9. NIH. (n.d.). Retrieved from Brain Basics: Understanding Sleep: www.ninds.nih.gov/Disorders/Patient-Caregiver-Education/ Understanding-Sleep

10. NIH. (n.d.). Retrieved from Brain Basics: Understanding Sleep: www.ninds.nih.gov/Disorders/Patient-Caregiver-Education/ Understanding-Sleep

11. NIH. (n.d.). Retrieved from Brain Basics: Understanding Sleep: www.ninds.nih.gov/Disorders/Patient-Caregiver-Education/ Understanding-Sleep

12. NIH. (n.d.). Retrieved from Brain Basics: Understanding Sleep: www.ninds.nih.gov/Disorders/Patient-Caregiver-Education/ Understanding-Sleep

13. Khandelwal, D., Dutta, D., Chittawar, S., & S, K. (2017, Sept-October). Sleep Disorders in Type 2 Diabetes. Indian Journal of Endocrinology and Metabolism, 758-761. Retrieved from Sleep Disorders in Type 2 Diabetes:
    https://www.ijem.in/article.asp?issn=2230-8210;year= 2017;volume=21;issue=5;spage=758;epage=761;aulast=Khandelwal

14. Khandelwal, D., Dutta, D., Chittawar, S., & S, K. (2017, Sept-October). Sleep Disorders in Type 2 Diabetes. Indian Journal of Endocrinology and Metabolism, 758-761. Retrieved from Sleep Disorders in Type 2 Diabetes:
    https://www.ijem.in/article.asp?issn=2230-8210;year= 2017;volume=21;issue=5;spage=758;epage=761;aulast=Khandelwal

15. Khandelwal, D., Dutta, D., Chittawar, S., & S, K. (2017, Sept-October). Sleep Disorders in Type 2 Diabetes. Indian Journal of Endocrinology and Metabolism, 758-761. Retrieved from Sleep Disorders in Type 2 Diabetes:
    https://www.ijem.in/article.asp?issn=2230-8210;year= 2017;volume=21;issue=5;spage=758;epage=761;aulast=Khandelwal
    Breus, M. (2018, May 8). The Sleep Doctor. Retrieved from Understanding The Connection Between Sleep And Diabetes: https://thesleepdoctor.com/2018/05/08/understanding-the-connection-between-sleep-and-diabetes/

16. Breus, M. (2018, May 8). The Sleep Doctor. Retrieved from Understanding The Connection Between Sleep And Diabetes:

https://thesleepdoctor.com/2018/05/08/understanding-the-connection-between-sleep-and-diabetes/

17. Breus, M. (2018, May 8). The Sleep Doctor. Retrieved from Understanding The Connection Between Sleep And Diabetes: https://thesleepdoctor.com/2018/05/08/understanding-the-connection-between-sleep-and-diabetes/

18. Khandelwal, D., Dutta, D., Chittawar, S., & S, K. (2017, Sept-October). Sleep Disorders in Type 2 Diabetes. Indian Journal of Endocrinology and Metabolism, 758-761. Retrieved from Sleep Disorders in Type 2 Diabetes:
    https://www.ijem.in/article.asp?issn=2230-8210;year=2017;volume=21;issue=5;spage=758;epage=761;aulast=Khandelwal

19. Chasens, E., & Luyster, F. (2016, February 29). Effect of Sleep Disturbances on Quality of Life, Diabetes Self-Care Behaviour, and Patient-Reported Outcomes. American Diabetes Association. Diabetes Spectrum, 20-23. Retrieved from https://spectrum.diabetesjournals.org/content/29/1/20

20. Editor. (2019, January 15). Diabetes.co.uk. Retrieved from Diabetes and Sleep: www.diabetes.co.uk/diabetes-and-sleep.html

21. Editor. (2019, January 15). Diabetes.co.uk. Retrieved from Diabetes and Sleep: www.diabetes.co.uk/diabetes-and-sleep.html

22. Editor. (2019, January 15). Diabetes.co.uk. Retrieved from Diabetes and Sleep: www.diabetes.co.uk/diabetes-and-sleep.html

23. Editor. (2019, January 15). Diabetes.co.uk. Retrieved from Diabetes and Sleep: www.diabetes.co.uk/diabetes-and-sleep.html

24. Breus, M. (2018, May 8). The Sleep Doctor. Retrieved from Understanding The Connection Between Sleep And Diabetes: https://thesleepdoctor.com/2018/05/08/understanding-the-connection-between-sleep-and-diabetes/

25. Pagano, R. (2017, January 7). Sleepline. Retrieved from Insulin and Sleep – Do Sleep Problems Cause Insulin Resistance?: www.sleepline.com/insulin

26. Breus, M. (2018, May 8). The Sleep Doctor. Retrieved from Understanding The Connection Between Sleep And Diabetes: https://thesleepdoctor.com/2018/05/08/understanding-the-connection-between-sleep-and-diabetes/

27. Breus, M. (2018, May 8). The Sleep Doctor. Retrieved from Understanding The Connection Between Sleep And Diabetes:

https://thesleepdoctor.com/2018/05/08/understanding-the-connection-between-sleep-and-diabetes/

28. Watson, S., & Cherney, K. (2020, May 15). Healthline. Retrieved from The Effects of Sleep Deprivation on Your Body: www.healthline.com/health/sleep-deprivation/effects-on-body

29. Watson, S., & Cherney, K. (2020, May 15). Healthline. Retrieved from The Effects of Sleep Deprivation on Your Body: www.healthline.com/health/sleep-deprivation/effects-on-body

30. Watson, S., & Cherney, K. (2020, May 15). Healthline. Retrieved from The Effects of Sleep Deprivation on Your Body: www.healthline.com/health/sleep-deprivation/effects-on-body

31. Watson, S., & Cherney, K. (2020, May 15). Healthline. Retrieved from The Effects of Sleep Deprivation on Your Body: www.healthline.com/health/sleep-deprivation/effects-on-body

32. Watson, S., & Cherney, K. (2020, May 15). Healthline. Retrieved from The Effects of Sleep Deprivation on Your Body: www.healthline.com/health/sleep-deprivation/effects-on-body

33. Watson, S., & Cherney, K. (2020, May 15). Healthline. Retrieved from The Effects of Sleep Deprivation on Your Body: www.healthline.com/health/sleep-deprivation/effects-on-body

34. Watson, S., & Cherney, K. (2020, May 15). Healthline. Retrieved from The Effects of Sleep Deprivation on Your Body: www.healthline.com/health/sleep-deprivation/effects-on-body

35. Harvard Health Publishing. (2012, July 1). Retrieved from 8 secrets to a good night's sleep: www.health.harvard.edu/sleep/8-secrets-to-a-good-nights-sleep

9. ADDRESSING MENTAL HEALTH: WHY REDUCING STRESS IS CRUCIAL

1. World Health Organization. (n.d.). Retrieved from Mental health in the Western Pacific: www.who.int/westernpacific/health-topics/mental-health

2. Writer, S. (2020, April 7). Reference. Retrieved from What Is the Psychological Definition of Stress? www.reference.com/worldview/psychological-definition-stress-7c6b1f8dbdcdf15

3. Good Thinking. (2020, June 5). Retrieved from Types of Stress: https://www.good-thinking.uk/types-stress

4. Good Thinking. (2020, June 5). Retrieved from Types of Stress: https://www.good-thinking.uk/types-stress

5. Good Thinking. (2020, June 5). Retrieved from Types of Stress: https://www.good-thinking.uk/types-stress

6. Scott, E. (2020, December 7). Very Well Mind. Retrieved from What Is Chronic Stress? https://www.verywellmind.com/chronic-stress-3145104

7. Schniederman, N., Ironson, G., & Siegel, S. (2004). STRESS AND HEALTH: Psychological, Behavioral, and Biological Determinants. Annual Review of Clinical Psychology, 607-628. Retrieved from: Psychological, Behavioral, and Biological Determinants: www.ncbi.nlm.nih.gov/pmc/articles/PMC2568977/

8. Schniederman, N., Ironson, G., & Siegel, S. (2004). STRESS AND HEALTH: Psychological, Behavioral, and Biological Determinants. Annual Review of Clinical Psychology, 607-628. Retrieved from: Psychological, Behavioral, and Biological Determinants: www.ncbi.nlm.nih.gov/pmc/articles/PMC2568977/

9. Schniederman, N., Ironson, G., & Siegel, S. (2004). STRESS AND HEALTH: Psychological, Behavioral, and Biological Determinants. Annual Review of Clinical Psychology, 607-628. Retrieved from: Psychological, Behavioral, and Biological Determinants: www.ncbi.nlm.nih.gov/pmc/articles/PMC2568977/

10. Schniederman, N., Ironson, G., & Siegel, S. (2004). STRESS AND HEALTH: Psychological, Behavioral, and Biological Determinants. Annual Review of Clinical Psychology, 607-628. Retrieved from: Psychological, Behavioral, and Biological Determinants: www.ncbi.nlm.nih.gov/pmc/articles/PMC2568977/

11. Schniederman, N., Ironson, G., & Siegel, S. (2004). STRESS AND HEALTH: Psychological, Behavioral, and Biological Determinants. Annual Review of Clinical Psychology, 607-628. Retrieved from: Psychological, Behavioral, and Biological Determinants: www.ncbi.nlm.nih.gov/pmc/articles/PMC2568977/

12. Yaribeygi, H., Panahi, Y., & Sahraei, H; et al (2017). The impact of stress on body function: A review. EXCLI Journal. Retrieved from www.excli.de/vol16/Sahebkar_Panahi_21072017_proof.pdf

13. Schniederman, N., Ironson, G., & Siegel, S. (2004). STRESS AND HEALTH: Psychological, Behavioral, and Biological Determinants. Annual Review of Clinical Psychology, 607-628. Retrieved from: Psychological, Behavioral, and Biological Determinants:

www.ncbi.nlm.nih.gov/pmc/articles/PMC2568977/

14. Yaribeygi, H., Panahi, Y., & Sahraei, H; et al (2017). The impact of stress on body function: A review. EXCLI Journal. Retrieved from www.excli.de/vol16/Sahebkar_Panahi_21072017_proof.pdf

15. Harris, M., Oldmeadow, C., & Hure, A, et al. (2017). tress increases the risk of type 2 diabetes onset in women: A 12-year longitudinal study using causal modeling. PLOS ONE. Retrieved from https://journals.plos.org/plosone/article?id=10.1371/journal.pone.0172126 Workplace Stress and MSDs: Current Thinking and Future: https://ergoweb.com/workplace-stress-and-msds-current-thinking-and-future-research/

16. Falco, G., Pirro, P., & Castelleno, E; et al (2015). The Relationship between Stress. Journal of Neurology and Psychology, 1-7. Retrieved from www.avensonline.org/wp-content/uploads/JNP-2332-3469-03-0018.pdf

17. Editor. (2019, January 15). Diabetes.co.uk. Retrieved from Diabetes and Stress: www.diabetes.co.uk/diabetes-destress.html

18. Caporuscio, J. (2019, August 30). How are diabetes and stress linked? Retrieved from Medical News Today: www.medicalnewstoday.com/articles/326193#summary

19. McEwen, B., & Sapolsky, R. (2006). Stress and Your Health. The Journal of Clinical Endocrinology & Metabolism, E2. Retrieved from https://academic.oup.com/jcem/article/91/2/E2/2843213

20. Lloyd, C., Smith, J., & Weinger, K (2005). Stress and Diabetes: A Review of the Links. American Diabetes Association, 121-127. Retrieved from https://spectrum.diabetesjournals.org/content/18/2/121

21. Understanding diabetes and mental health. (n.d.). Retrieved from American Diabetes Association: https://www.diabetes.org/healthy-living/mental-health

22. Geer, K. (2020, April 16). Is Stress the Source of Your Blood Sugar Swing? Retrieved from Everyday Health: www.everydayhealth.com/hs/type-2-diabetes-management/stress-blood-sugar-swing

23. Sullivan, D. (2020, May 29). Stress: How It Affects Diabetes and How to Decrease It. Retrieved from Healthline: www.healthline.com/health/diabetes-and-stress

10. IF YOU HAVEN'T ALREADY, NOW'S THE TIME TO STOP SMOKING

1. Chang, S. (2012). Smoking and Type 2 Diabetes Mellitus. Diabetes and Metabolism Journal, 399-403. Retrieved from www.e-dmj.org/journal/view.php?doi=10.4093/dmj.2012.36.6.399

2. Ambrose, J., & R, B. (2004). The Pathophysiology of Cigarette Smoking and Cardiovascular Disease: An update. Journal of the American College of Cardiology, 1737-1737. Retrieved from www.sciencedirect.com/science/article/pii/S0735109704004346

3. Paula. (2016, July 2). Describe the contents of smoked tobacco in terms of the particulate and gaseous phases. Retrieved from science: https://sciemce.com/956489/describe-contents-smoked-tobacco-particulate-gaseous-phases

4. Berkowitz, L., Schultz, B., & Salazar, G. (2018, January 30). Impact of Cigarette Smoking on the Gastrointestinal Tract Inflammation: Opposing Effects in Crohn's Disease and Ulcerative Colitis. Retrieved from Frontiers in Immunology: www.frontiersin.org/articles/10.3389/fimmu.2018.00074/full

5. Berkowitz, L., Schultz, B., & Salazar, G. (2018, January 30). Impact of Cigarette Smoking on the Gastrointestinal Tract Inflammation: Opposing Effects in Crohn's Disease and Ulcerative Colitis. Retrieved from Frontiers in Immunology: www.frontiersin.org/articles/10.3389/fimmu.2018.00074/full

6. Arshad, H. (n.d.). SlideShare. Retrieved from Pathological Effects of Smoking: https://www.slideshare.net/xubiaarshad3/pathological-effects-of-smoking

7. Ambrose, J., & R, B. (2004). The Pathophysiology of Cigarette Smoking and Cardiovascular Disease: An update. Journal of the American College of Cardiology, 1737-1737. Retrieved from www.sciencedirect.com/science/article/pii/S0735109704004346

8. Arshad, H. (n.d.). SlideShare. Retrieved from Pathological Effects of Smoking: https://www.slideshare.net/xubiaarshad3/pathological-effects-of-smoking

9. Berkowitz, L., Schultz, B., & Salazar, G. (2018, January 30). Impact of Cigarette Smoking on the Gastrointestinal Tract Inflammation: Opposing Effects in Crohn's Disease and Ulcerative Colitis.

Retrieved from Frontiers in Immunology: www.frontiersin.org/
articles/10.3389/fimmu.2018.00074/full

10. Arshad, H. (n.d.). SlideShare. Retrieved from Pathological Effects of
Smoking: https://www.slideshare.net/xubiaarshad3/pathological-
effects-of-smoking

11. Berkowitz, L., Schultz, B., & Salazar, G. (2018, January 30). Impact
of Cigarette Smoking on the Gastrointestinal Tract Inflammation:
Opposing Effects in Crohn's Disease and Ulcerative Colitis.
Retrieved from Frontiers in Immunology: www.frontiersin.org/
articles/10.3389/fimmu.2018.00074/full

12. Tweed, J., Hsia, S., Lufty, K., Friedman, TC (2012). The Endocrine
Effects of Nicotine and Cigarette smoke. Trends in Endocrinology
and Metabolism, 334-342. https://doi.org/10.1016/j.tem.2012.
03.006

13. Lindberg, S. (2019, August 23). What You Need to Know About
Smoking and Your Brain. Retrieved from Healthline: www.
healthline.com/health/smoking/smoking-effects-on-brain

14. Lande, R. (2018, July 16). Nicotine Addiction. Retrieved from
Medscape:
https://emedicine.medscape.com/article/287555-overview#a3

15. Tweed, J., Hsia, S., Lufty, K., Friedman, TC (2012). The Endocrine
Effects of Nicotine and Cigarette smoke. Trends in Endocrinology
and Metabolism, 334-342. https://doi.org/10.1016/j.tem.2012.
03.006

16. Tweed, J., Hsia, S., Lufty, K., Friedman, TC (2012). The Endocrine
Effects of Nicotine and Cigarette smoke. Trends in Endocrinology
and Metabolism, 334-342. https://doi.org/10.1016/j.tem.2012.
03.006

17. Tweed, J., Hsia, S., Lufty, K., Friedman, TC (2012). The Endocrine
Effects of Nicotine and Cigarette smoke. Trends in Endocrinology
and Metabolism, 334-342. https://doi.org/10.1016/j.tem.2012.
03.006

18. Chang, S. (2012). Smoking and Type 2 Diabetes Mellitus. Diabetes
and Metabolism Journal, 399-403. Retrieved from www.e-dmj.org/
journal/view.php?doi=10.4093/dmj.2012.36.6.399

19. Tweed, J., Hsia, S., Lufty, K., Friedman, TC (2012). The Endocrine
Effects of Nicotine and Cigarette smoke. Trends in Endocrinology
and Metabolism, 334-342. https://doi.org/10.1016/j.tem.2012.
03.006

20. Chang, S. (2012). Smoking and Type 2 Diabetes Mellitus. Diabetes and Metabolism Journal, 399-403. Retrieved from www.e-dmj.org/journal/view.php?doi=10.4093/dmj.2012.36.6.399

21. Tweed, J., Hsia, S., Lufty, K., Friedman, TC (2012). The Endocrine Effects of Nicotine and Cigarette smoke. Trends in Endocrinology and Metabolism, 334-342. https://doi.org/10.1016/j.tem.2012.03.006

22. Tilg, H., & Moschen, A. (2008). Insulin resistance, inflammation, and non-alcoholic fatty liver disease. Trends in Endocrinology and Metabolism, 371-379. https://doi.org/10.1016/j.tem.2008.08.005

23. Tweed, J., Hsia, S., Lufty, K., Friedman, TC (2012). The Endocrine Effects of Nicotine and Cigarette smoke. Trends in Endocrinology and Metabolism, 334-342. https://doi.org/10.1016/j.tem.2012.03.006

24. Tweed, J., Hsia, S., Lufty, K., Friedman, TC (2012). The Endocrine Effects of Nicotine and Cigarette smoke. Trends in Endocrinology and Metabolism, 334-342. https://doi.org/10.1016/j.tem.2012.03.006

25. Tweed, J., Hsia, S., Lufty, K., Friedman, TC (2012). The Endocrine Effects of Nicotine and Cigarette smoke. Trends in Endocrinology and Metabolism, 334-342. https://doi.org/10.1016/j.tem.2012.03.006

26. Tweed, J., Hsia, S., Lufty, K., Friedman, TC (2012). The Endocrine Effects of Nicotine and Cigarette smoke. Trends in Endocrinology and Metabolism, 334-342. https://doi.org/10.1016/j.tem.2012.03.006

27. Chang, S. (2012). Smoking and Type 2 Diabetes Mellitus. Diabetes and Metabolism Journal, 399-403. Retrieved from www.e-dmj.org/journal/view.php?doi=10.4093/dmj.2012.36.6.399

28. Villines, Z. (2021, January 14). How does smoking affect the risk of diabetes? Retrieved from MedicalNewsToday: www.medicalnewstoday.com/articles/317411#lowering-the-risk

29. Villines, Z. (2021, January 14). How does smoking affect the risk of diabetes? Retrieved from MedicalNewsToday: www.medicalnewstoday.com/articles/317411#lowering-the-risk

30. Villines, Z. (2021, January 14). How does smoking affect the risk of diabetes? Retrieved from MedicalNewsToday: www.medicalnewstoday.com/articles/317411#lowering-the-risk

31. Villines, Z. (2021, January 14). How does smoking affect the risk of diabetes? Retrieved from MedicalNewsToday: www.medicalnewstoday.com/articles/317411#lowering-the-risk

32. Gometz, E. (2011). Health Effects of Smoking and the Benefits of Quitting. AMA Journal of Ethics, 31-35. Retrieved from https://journalofethics.ama-assn.org/article/health-effects-smoking-and-benefits-quitting/2011-01

33. Villines, Z. (2021, January 14). How does smoking affect the risk of diabetes? Retrieved from MedicalNewsToday: www.medicalnewstoday.com/articles/317411#lowering-the-risk

34. Villines, Z. (2021, January 14). How does smoking affect the risk of diabetes? Retrieved from MedicalNewsToday: www.medicalnewstoday.com/articles/317411#lowering-the-risk

35. Villines, Z. (2021, January 14). How does smoking affect the risk of diabetes? Retrieved from MedicalNewsToday: www.medicalnewstoday.com/articles/317411#lowering-the-risk

36. Villines, Z. (2021, January 14). How does smoking affect the risk of diabetes? Retrieved from MedicalNewsToday: www.medicalnewstoday.com/articles/317411#lowering-the-risk; Gometz, E. (2011). Health Effects of Smoking and the Benefits of Quitting. AMA Journal of Ethics, 31-35. Retrieved from https://journalofethics.ama-assn.org/article/health-effects-smoking-and-benefits-quitting/2011-01

37. Gometz, E. (2011). Health Effects of Smoking and the Benefits of Quitting. AMA Journal of Ethics, 31-35. Retrieved from https://journalofethics.ama-assn.org/article/health-effects-smoking-and-benefits-quitting/2011-01

38. What is Nicotine Withdrawal? (n.d.). Retrieved from WebMD: www.webmd.com/smoking-cessation/understanding-nicotine-withdrawal-symptoms

39. Villines, Z. (2021, January 14). How does smoking affect the risk of diabetes? Retrieved from MedicalNewsToday: www.medicalnewstoday.com/articles/317411#lowering-the-risk

www.ingramcontent.com/pod-product-compliance
Lightning Source LLC
Chambersburg PA
CBHW010246030426
42336CB00022B/3317